Arthrodesis of the Foot and Ankle

Guest Editors

STEVEN F. BOC, DPM
VINCENT MUSCARELLA, DPM

CLINICS IN PODIATRIC MEDICINE AND SURGERY

www.podiatric.theclinics.com

Consulting Editor
THOMAS ZGONIS, DPM, FACFAS

January 2012 • Volume 29 • Number 1

SAUNDERS an imprint of ELSEVIER, Inc.

W.B. SAUNDERS COMPANY
A Division of Elsevier Inc.

1600 John F. Kennedy Boulevard • Suite 1800 • Philadelphia, Pennsylvania 19103-2899

http://www.theclinics.com

CLINICS IN PODIATRIC MEDICINE AND SURGERY Volume 29, Number 1
January 2012 ISSN 0891-8422, ISBN-13: 978-1-4557-3921-9

Editor: Patrick Manley

Clinics in Podiatric Medicine and Surgery (ISSN 0891-8422) is published quarterly by Elsevier Inc., 360 Park Avenue South, New York, NY 10010-1710. Months of issue are January, April, July, and October. Business and Editorial Offices: 1600 John F. Kennedy Blvd., Ste. 1800, Philadelphia, PA 19103-2899. Customer Service Office: 3251 Riverport Lane, Maryland Heights, MO 63043. Periodicals postage paid at NewYork, NY and additional mailing offices. Subscription prices are $292.00 per year for US individuals, $410.00 per year for US institutions, $148.00 per year for US students and residents, $350.00 per year for Canadian individuals, $508.00 for Canadian institutions, $415.00 for international individuals, $508.00 per year for international institutions and $208.00 per year for Canadian and foreign students/residents. To receive student/resident rate, orders must be accompanied by name of affiliated institution, date of term, and the *signature* of program/residency coordinator on institution letterhead. Orders will be billed at individual rate until proof of status is received. Foreign air speed delivery is included in all *Clinics* subscription prices. All prices are subject to change without notice. POSTMASTER: Send address changes to *Clinics in Podiatric Medicine and Surgery*, Elsevier Health Sciences Division, Subscription Customer Service, 3251 Riverport Lane, Maryland Heights, MO 63043. **Customer Service: 1-800-654-2452 (US). From outside of the US, call 314-447-8871. Fax: 314-447-8029. E-mail: JournalsCustomerService-usa@elsevier.com (for print support); JournalsOnlineSupport-usa@elsevier.com (for online support).**

Reprints. For copies of 100 or more of articles in this publication, please contact the Commercial Reprints Department, Elsevier Inc., 360 Park Avenue South, New York, NY 10010-1710. Tel.: 212-633-3812; Fax: 212-462-1935; E-mail: reprints@elsevier.com.

Clinics in Podiatric Medicine and Surgery is covered in *MEDLINE/PubMed (Index Medicus) and EMBASE/Excerpta Medica.*

Printed and bound by CPI Group (UK) Ltd, Croydon, CR0 4YY

Transferred to Digital Print 2012

Contributors

CONSULTING EDITOR

THOMAS ZGONIS, DPM, FACFAS
Associate Professor, Reconstructive Foot and Ankle Fellowship Director and Chief, Division of Podiatric Medicine and Surgery, Department of Orthopedic Surgery, The University of Texas Health Science Center at San Antonio, San Antonio, Texas

GUEST EDITORS

STEVEN F. BOC, DPM, FACFAS, FACFOAM
Director of Resident Training, Podiatric Medicine and Surgery Program, Hahnemann University Hospital; Clinical Associate Professor, Department of Surgery, Drexel College of Medicine, Hahnemann University Hospital, Philadelphia, Pennsylvania

VINCENT MUSCARELLA, DPM, FACFAS
Department of Surgery, Drexel College of Medicine Hahnemann University Hospital, Philadelphia, Pennsylvania

AUTHORS

NEDA ARJOMANDI, MS, DPM
Third Year Podiatric Medicine and Surgery Resident, Kennedy Memorial Hospital, University Medical Center, Stratford, New Jersey

SAMANTHA BANGA, DPM
Podiatric Medicine and Surgery Resident, Hahnemann University Hospital, Drexel University College of Medicine, Philadelphia, Pennsylvania

MOHSEN BARMADA, DPM
PGY2, Hahnemann University Hospital, Philadelphia, Pennsylvania

JADE BARNARD, DPM
Resident, Podiatric Medicine and Surgery, Kennedy University Hospital, Stratford, New Jersey

STEVEN F. BOC, DPM, FACFAS, FACFOAM
Director of Resident Training, Podiatric Medicine and Surgery Program, Hahnemann University Hospital; Clinical Associate Professor, Department of Surgery, Drexel College of Medicine, Hahnemann University Hospital, Philadelphia, Pennsylvania

ALBERT M. D'ANGELANTONIO, BSME, DPM, FACFAS
Director, Podiatric Medicine and Surgery, Kennedy University Hospital, Stratford; Private Practice, Regional Foot and Ankle Specialists, Turnersville, New Jersey

CRYSTAL N. GONZALEZ, DPM
Attending, Associate, Allentown Family Foot Care, PC, Lehigh Valley Health Network, St Luke's Health Network, Sacred Heart Hospital, Macungie, Pennsylvania

NAFISA HASAN, DPM
Podiatric Medicine and Surgery Resident, Hahnemann University Hospital, Drexel University College of Medicine, Philadelphia, Pennsylvania

STEVEN KISSEL, DPM
Podiatric Surgical Resident, Division of Podiatric Medicine and Surgery, Department of Orthopaedic Surgery, University of Texas Health Science Center at San Antonio, San Antonio, Texas

NADIA LEVY, DPM
Senior Resident in Podiatric Surgery, Saint Francis Hospital and Medical Center, Hartford, Connecticut

RAMON LOPEZ, DPM
Diplomate, The American Board of Podiatric Surgery; Diplomate, The American Board of Podiatric Orthopedics and Primary Podiatric Medicine; Hahnemann University Hospital, Drexel University College of Medicine, Philadelphia; Horsham Foot and Ankle Group, Horsham, Pennsylvania

JEFFREY MARTONE, DPM
Adjunct Clinical Professor of Podiatric Surgery, Temple University School of Medicine, Philadelphia, Pennsylvania; Barry University, Miami Shores, Florida; Rosalind Franklin University, Dr William M. Scholl School of Podiatric Medicine, Illinois; Attending Staff, Private Practice, Department of Surgery, Saint Francis Hospital and Medical Center, East Hartford, Connecticut

PATRICK R. MCDONALD, DPM
Former PGY3, Hahnemann University Hospital; Private Practice, Orthopedics, P.C, Pennsylvania

VINCENT MUSCARELLA, DPM, FACFAS
Department of Surgery, Drexel College of Medicine Hahnemann University Hospital, Philadelphia, Pennsylvania

KAITLIN A. NELSON-RINALDI, DPM
Chief Resident, Podiatric Medicine and Surgery, Kennedy University Hospital, Stratford, New Jersey

NATHAN D. NOREM, DPM
PGY-III and Chief Resident, Foot and Ankle Surgical Residency Program, Hahnemann University Hospital/Drexel University College of Medicine, Philadelphia, Pennsylvania

FRANK OWARE, DPM
Podiatric Medicine and Surgery, Kennedy University Hospital, Stratford, New Jersey

PANAGIOTIS PANAGAKOS, DPM, AACFAS
Attending, Associate, Foot and Ankle Care Associates, LLC, Attending, Hahnemann University Hospital, Overlook Hospital, Staten Island, New York

KRUPA PATEL, DPM, AACFAS
Associate, Foot and Ankle Specialists of New Jersey, Westfield, New Jersey

LAURA VANDER POEL, DPM
Senior Resident in Podiatric Surgery, Saint Francis Hospital and Medical Center, Hartford, Connecticut

JOSEPH PUSATERI, DPM
PGY-1 Hahneman University Hospital, Podiatric Medicine and Surgery Residency Program, Philadelphia, Pennsylvania

ROBERT M. RAJCZY, DPM
PGY2, Hahnemann University Hospital, Philadelphia, Pennsylvania

CRYSTAL L. RAMANUJAM, DPM, MSc
Assistant Professor, Division of Podiatric Medicine and Surgery, Department of Orthopaedic Surgery, University of Texas Health Science Center at San Antonio, San Antonio, Texas

SOORENA SADRI, DPM
Chief Resident, Hahnemann University Hospital, Podiatric Medicine and Surgery Residency Program, Philadelphia, Pennsylvania

FAITH A. SCHICK, DPM
Medical Staff, Community Medical Center; Private Practice, Toms River, New Jersey

HOWARD S. SHAPIRO, DPM
Assistant Director of Residency and Podiatric Education, Hahnemann University Hospital, Podiatric Medicine Surgery Program, Philadelphia, Pennsylvania

TARIKA SINGH, DPM, AACFAS
The Foot and Ankle Group, P.C. Aria Health, Philadelphia, Pennsylvania

ALEX STEWART, DPM
Podiatric Surgical Resident, Division of Podiatric Medicine and Surgery, Department of Orthopaedic Surgery, University of Texas Health Science Center at San Antonio, San Antonio, Texas

NATHAN ULLOM, DPM
Department of Podiatric Medical Education, Podiatric Medicine and Surgery Resident, Hahnemann University Hospital, Philadelphia, Pennsylvania

THOMAS ZGONIS, DPM, FACFAS
Associate Professor, Reconstructive Foot and Ankle Fellowship Director and Chief, Division of Podiatric Medicine and Surgery, Department of Orthopedic Surgery, The University of Texas Health Science Center at San Antonio, San Antonio, Texas

Contents

motion is noted at the joint. Arthrodesis at the first MTPJ also has it uses as a primary procedure for rheumatoid arthritis when severe deformity is present, as well as for salvage procedures for failed joint arthroplasties with or without implant, fractures with intra-articular extension, avascular necrosis, and infection management. A first MTPJ arthrodesis should provide stable fixation, attain suitable positioning for a reasonable gait, maintain adequate length, and create a stable platform for a plantigrade foot type.

Lisfranc fracture-dislocations are complex injuries that require a high skill set from foot and ankle surgeons to diagnose and treat. Conservative treatment is seldom an option for treatment of Lisfranc injuries. The authors believe that even subtle injuries require surgical intervention. The comparison between open reduction internal fixation, partial arthrodesis, and complete arthrodesis is discussed, as well as various fixation techniques to accomplish these procedures when approaching a Lisfranc injury.

Isolated subtalar joint arthrodesis has gained popularity more recently. Research has shown that it preserves rearfoot motion, does not increase the risk of arthritis in adjacent joints, and is not an especially complex operative procedure. It decreases the chance of midtarsal joint nonunion and malunion postoperatively. This article takes an in-depth approach to isolated talocalcaneal fusions. Anatomy and biomechanics of the subtalar joint are reviewed. Clinical presentation and radiologic evaluation are discussed. Conservative treatment, operative technique, and postoperative management are included.

The calcaneocuboid joint is stable, although multiple conditions might affect the joint, including arthritis, fracture, subluxation, and dislocation. Calcaneocuboid arthrodesis is more commonly performed as an adjunct procedure with other rearfoot procedures such as triple arthrodesis and is less used as isolated fusion. This article reviews the main conditions of the lateral column and calcaneocuboid joint in particular. The surgical technique for isolated calcaneocuboid arthrodesis is discussed.

A triple arthrodesis is a fusion of the talocalcaneal, calcaneal cuboid, and talonavicular joints. The purpose is to create a well-aligned, plantigrade, and stable foot for patients with deformity or progressive neurologic and arthritic conditions. This article is a comprehensive overview of the procedure. However effective, triple arthrodesis is a challenging procedure for even the most skilled surgeon.

This article presents an overview of current ankle arthrodesis techniques. Surgical indications, pathophysiology of the ankle joint, preoperative assessment of the patient, surgical techniques for ankle fusion, and complications/sequelae are discussed. The surgical techniques section focuses on crossed screws arthrodesis and intramedullary nailing for tibiotalocalcaneal arthrodesis. Other techniques, including arthroscopic fusion, are also discussed.

The principles of fusion of a Charcot joint arise from the assertion that successful fusion requires removal of all cartilage, debris, and sclerotic bone. The authors believe that reconstruction can prevent amputation in patients who have unbraceable or unstable deformities, or recurrent ulcerations. The goal with any Charcot reconstruction procedure is to achieve a plantigrade foot free of ulceration, and to prevent any future collapse, deformity, or ulcerations. The authors strongly believe arthrodesis of unstable joints of the Charcot neuropathic foot can lead to limb salvage and better quality of life.

Current Concepts and Techniques in Foot and Ankle Surgery

The primary goal in the treatment of arthritic joints is elimination of pain associated with limited motion. Several surgical techniques have been developed to treat varying degrees of hallux rigidus of any cause. This case report details an alternative surgical approach to address hallux rigidus and associated hallux valgus deformity through a combination of joint debridement, resurfacing, and arthrodiastasis.

Creative surgical strategies are often warranted for long-term closure of diabetic foot wounds. This article provides a case report describing the successive use of negative pressure wound therapy, advanced biologics, and split thickness skin grafting for healing an extensive surgical wound. Although the success of these therapies is enticing, their use should be based on careful patient selection in a multidisciplinary setting.

THE CLINICS ARE NOW AVAILABLE ONLINE!

Access your subscription at:
www.theclinics.com

Foreword

Arthrodesis of the Foot and Ankle

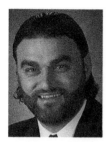

Thomas Zgonis, DPM
Consulting Editor

The powerful outcome of arthrodesis for the management of various foot and ankle pathologies is being studied continuously through biomechanical and clinical research. The gratifying result of a successful arthrodesis and alignment along with the unforgiving possible sequela of a nonunion and/or malunion still exists in every surgeon's mind each time the procedure is performed.

The role of arthrodesis to address painful and debilitating foot and ankle conditions is numerous to say the least. While the topic is broad, the selected authors have addressed the indications, techniques, and pearls along with key insights on postoperative protocols to avoid potential complications. The guest editors Drs Boc and Muscarella have done an outstanding job on their contributions and by selecting surgical experts to collaborate for the making of this edition.

Through continuous education, teaching, and research, we are able to improve outcomes for those individuals who require a successful arthrodesis procedure. Even though the incidence of nonunion may be low in most elective foot and ankle procedures, further technological and biological advances are already in motion to complement sound surgical techniques and skills when performing an arthrodesis. This edition not only demonstrates the new advances in arthrodesis procedures of the foot and ankle but also emphasizes the importance of surgical experience and training to improve our surgical outcomes.

Thomas Zgonis, DPM
Division of Podiatric Medicine and Surgery
Department of Orthopaedic Surgery
The University of Texas Health Science Center at San Antonio
7703 Floyd Curl Drive–MSC 7776
San Antonio, TX 78229, USA

E-mail address:
zgonis@uthscsa.edu

Clin Podiatr Med Surg 29 (2012) xiii
doi:10.1016/j.cpm.2011.12.001
0891-8422/12/$ – see front matter © 2012 Elsevier Inc. All rights reserved.

Preface

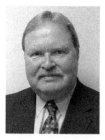 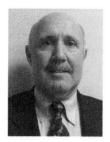

Steven F. Boc, DPM   Vincent Muscarella, DPM
Guest Editors

My colleagues and I appreciate the honor and opportunity to participate in writing various articles for *Clinics in Podiatric Medicine and Surgery*, undertaking the extensive and broad-range topic of arthrodesis of the foot and ankle. Serving as a guest editor, I recognize the ultimate responsibility to provide a thorough and comprehensive review and inclusion of various topics on arthrodesis that would be relevant to foot and ankle surgeons. Arthrodesis can be a technically complex procedure in inexperienced hands. The ultimate decision to perform arthrodesis procedures is contingent on the need to perform salvage procedures due to a patient's continued pain and disability after alternative treatments have failed.

I am fortunate enough to have an association with a high-caliber group of surgeons in the Philadelphia area; many of whom have worked together closely through the years at major teaching institutions. I am also privileged to be a mentor and train a highly talented group of residents at the Hahnemann University Hospital residency program. All of the authors have had the opportunity to learn first and then teach arthrodesis techniques to their colleagues and peers.

The authors have contributed topics to cover fusion techniques employing various types of fixation from the digits through the mid foot, including the rear foot and ankle. In addition, Charcot reconstruction, as well as various salvage techniques, was employed to provide a comprehensive review of the pathology that confronts lower extremity surgeons.

No text or article is authoritative in and by itself. By utilizing the information of many physicians and surgeons, and the current literature available, the individual surgeon can make a rational decision that is appropriate in the management and salvage of patients with significant deformities. I hope the readers of these various articles will take into consideration the thought and effort that went into the compilation of information and recognize that this is just a stepping stone for them to have an understanding of various arthrodesis techniques. The reader should be able to take the information provided, expound on it, and assure the best outcomes for their patients.

Clin Podiatr Med Surg 29 (2012) xv–xvi
doi:10.1016/j.cpm.2011.12.002
0891-8422/12/$ – see front matter © 2012 Elsevier Inc. All rights reserved.

Without a doubt, surgical experience, interaction with peers, case trial and error, research, and review of available materials are all part of the surgical armament when designing and performing arthrodesis techniques.

I thank all of those who participated in making this endeavor possible, including Dr Zgonis and the surgical faculty, many of whom I've worked with at either Metropolitan Hospital, St Agnes Hospital, or Hahnemann University Hospital in Philadelphia.

Steven F. Boc, DPM
Vincent Muscarella, DPM

Department of Surgery, Drexel College of Medicine/
Hahnemann University Hospital
235 North Broad Street
Philadelphia, PA 19107, USA

E-mail addresses:
Sfbocdpm1@comcast.net (S.F. Boc)
vmuscarella@comcast.net (V. Muscarella)

Indications and Considerations of Foot and Ankle Arthrodesis

Vincent Muscarella, DPM, Soorena Sadri, DPM*,
Joseph Pusateri, DPM

KEYWORDS

- Arthrodesis • Foot and ankle complex • Bone healing
- Foot and ankle biomechanics

CONSIDERATIONS AND INDICATIONS OF FOOT AND ANKLE ARTHRODESIS

The foot and ankle of the human body is a complex system of integrated units composed of bones, tendons, muscles, and ligaments. Like a well-oiled machine, each part must move and react in perfect harmony. The joints of the foot and ankle can suffer many trials and tribulations in an otherwise normal human life. The foot and ankle at times must adapt to these instances, from fractures and dislocations to congenital problems. When adaptation leads to a malformation in the unit structure, surgical intervention is required to restore the foot and ankle complex to a working device.

As foot and ankle surgeons, our responsibility lies in restoring the foot and ankle to a relatively pain-free structure. Primary indications for regarding any joint fusion in the human body include deformity, instability and, more importantly, pain. Fusions involving single and multiple joints are indicated for a myriad of conditions including primary osteoarthritis, posttraumatic arthritis, neoplasms, malunion, nonunion, congenital anomalies, and neurotraumatic injury.

This article gives an overview of the indications for performing joint fusions at the foot and ankle.

JOINTS OF THE FOOT AND ANKLE

To begin the discussion of indications of foot and ankle arthrodesis, a review of what constitutes a joint is needed. A joint or articulation is the union of 2 or more bones, allowing transmission of forces (shear, compressive, and torsion), differential growth,

The Foot and Ankle Center of Philadelphia, Hahnemann University Hospital/Drexel University College of Medicine, Podiatric Medicine and Surgery Residency Program, 235 North Broad Street, Suite 300, Philadelphia, PA, USA
* Corresponding author.
E-mail address: drsoorenasadri@gmail.com

Clin Podiatr Med Surg 29 (2012) 1–9
doi:10.1016/j.cpm.2011.09.001
0891-8422/12/$ – see front matter © 2012 Elsevier Inc. All rights reserved.

and movement. Two classification schemes designed to describe joints have been developed. The amount of movement between the bones and the type of connection between the joints has been described. The traditional classification scheme describing movement between joints is divided into synarthrosis, amphiarthrosis, and diarthrosis. Synarthrosis joints in the foot and ankle include the tibiofibular joint, joints that provide very little movement. Amphiarthrosis joints are those such as the calcaneocuboid joint or the metatarsal cuneiform joints, which allow greater flexibility but are connected by fibrocartilage. Joints that permit free movement between bones are classified as a diarthrosis or synovial joint.[1]

A modification of the aforementioned joint classification scheme is based on the type of connection between bones rather than the amount of movement involved. In the foot and ankle there are several examples of such joints. The interphalangeal joints are described as hinge or ginglymus joints. The bones that provide this motion have trochlear articular shapes at the facets, are reinforced with collateral ligaments on each side, and provide one axis of motion, mainly flexion and extension. The ankle joint is a modified hinge joint in that the majority of its motion lies in the sagittal plane with slight motion of the transverse plane occurring as well.[2] The metatarsophalangeal joints are described as ellipsoid or condyloid joints. The bones that provide this motion have facets that are concave that rotate on an oval head that is much greater in length than width. Metatarsophalangeal joints have 2 axes of motion, adduction and abduction on the short axis and flexion and extension on the long axis. The calcaneocuboid joint is described as a saddle or sellar joint in which the facets have a saddle shape and one side of the facet is turned down. The calcaneocuboid joint has 2 axes of motion; however, motion at this joint is very limited, due to the strong ligaments surrounding this joint. The talonavicular joint is described as a ball and socket or enarthrodial joint, which allows circumduction as well as allowing 3 axes of motion.

COMPOSITION OF JOINT STRUCTURES

The joints of the foot and ankle are surrounded by a great synovial lining called the great tarsal cavity. Each joint surface is covered by varying thickness of articular cartilage. Joint contact is limited between these cartilaginous surfaces, resulting in a low coefficient of friction. Synovial fluid bathes these surfaces and acts like a lubricant. The synovial fluid is also involved in maintenance of living cells in the articular cartilage. Articular cartilage has a slightly compressible and elastic surface. This configuration allows it to be able to absorb the large compressive forces generated by movement across these surfaces. Thickness of articular cartilage ranges from 1 to 2 mm. There is an age difference in the appearance of articular cartilage; in youth it tends to be compressible whereas in aged individuals it tends to be brittle with an irregular surface. Articular cartilage is molded to the joint surfaces and varies in thickness depending on the surface. Concave articular cartilages are thinnest centrally and thicker peripherally, and convex articular cartilages are thickest centrally while thinning peripherally. The peripheral vascular plexus in the synovial membrane is said to provide nutrition to the articular cartilages. Also, articular cartilage has no blood vessels or nerve supply. With increasing age, the articular cartilage will develop wear and tear in the form of jagged edges and small debris within the synovial joint.[3]

Synovial membrane secretes synovial fluid. Synovial membrane is derived from embryonic mesenchyme and covers all nonarticular areas where movement occurs between surfaces. Specifically in joints, it lines the intracapsular ligaments, tendon sheaths, and fibrous capsules. It does not line the articular cartilage; there is a structural transition zone between the articular cartilage and the synovial membrane.

Articular fat pads are accumulations of adipose tissue that occur in synovial membranes in joints. Articular fat pads occupy the irregularities and potential spaces in joints and when the joint undergoes motion to accommodate to the changing shape and volume of the irregularities. The fat pads allow the distribution of synovial fluid over articular surfaces. Synovial villi line the internal synovial membrane. These villi rest near articular margins and increase with age, which can become a factor in the majority of pathologic joint dysfunction.

MECHANISM OF BONE HEALING

Understanding the biology of bone healing is paramount to the understanding of correct arthrodesis techniques for the foot and ankle surgeon. As part of the surgeon's armamentarium of understanding, knowing the basic biology of bone can be to the surgeon's advantage and can prove beneficial in the surgical theater.

A mineralized version of connective tissue, bone, is unique in that it allows for scarless tissue regeneration provided the bone is reapproximated in an anatomic fashion. Bone is formed by cells called osteoblasts. These osteoblasts deposit a type-I collagen matrix that releases magnesium, calcium, and phosphate ions, which form a matrix in the form of hydroxyapatite. The composition of bone is twofold, being composed of a hard mineral and a flexible collagen matrix, which makes it stronger and harder than cartilage. These two properties prevent the structure of bone from being brittle, unlike cartilage, which can become quite brittle over time.[4]

The functional unit of bone is the osteon, which consists of a Haversian canal system containing blood and nerve supply. The osteon contains concentric layers of mineralized matrix called concentric lamellae. Two types of osseous tissue are spongy and compact. Spongy bone encompasses the hollow interior while compact bone consists of the hard exterior.

Of importance is that bone tissue and bone are two different entities. Bone tissue is a type of connective tissue that is specifically made of the mineral matrix whereas bones are structures made up of bone tissue, marrow, nerves, blood vessels, and epithelium. Cortical bone studies have shown that bone has poor tensile strength of approximately 133 MPa in the longitudinal plane and 51.0 MPa in the transverse plane, and a low shear stress strength of 51.6 MPa.[5] However, bone has a relatively high compressive strength of 193 MPa in the longitudinal plane and 133 MPa in the transverse plane.[6] These results clearly show that the compressive strength of bone is much greater than the tension and shear strength.

An understanding of the basics of fracture healing is paramount to the fundamental principles of arthrodesis. Fracture healing is divided into two types, direct and indirect healing. Direct fracture healing or primary fracture healing is performed by internal remodeling and occurs only with absolute stability, and is the process of osteonal bone remodeling.[4] Indirect or secondary healing occurs with relative stability and is performed by callus formation. Arthrodesis principles require that the patient undergo primary healing of bone. Because of the high incidence of nonunion in arthrodesis procedures, secondary bone healing must and should be prevented.

Regardless of the type of bone healing involved, both primary and secondary healing undergo 4 basic stages: inflammation, soft callus formation, hard callus formation, and remodeling.[7] The inflammatory stage begins rapidly and continues until formation of cartilage, fibrous tissue, or bone begins. This phase takes place from 1 to 7 days after the initial fracture has occurred. At first there is inflammatory exudation from damaged blood vessels and hematoma formation. At the ends of the fracture bone necrosis occurs. Embedded in this hematoma is a dense network of reticulin fibrils, fibrin, collagen, and cytokines that produces vasodilatation to the surrounding tissues. The formation of fracture hematoma gradually is replaced by granulation tissue. The bone fragment ends, although minimal in primary healing, begin to become resorbed by osteoclasts that remove the necrotic ends of bone.

The next stage, soft callus formation, brings a decrease in pain and swelling and corresponds to the immovable free ends of the bone fracture. This stage takes place approximately 2 to 3 weeks postfracture. Unfortunately, while the stability of the soft callus stage is adequate to prevent shortening, angulation at the site of fracture may still occur, leading to a malalignment of the fracture ends. The characteristic property of the soft callus stage is growth of callus. Osteoblasts are created from the cells in the periosteum and endosteum. The fracture ends slowly bridge and link together to form a soft callus with a combination of chondrocytes and fibroblasts.

The hard callus formation stage begins when the soft callus links the two bone ends together. The soft callus within the gap undergoes endochondral bone formation, and the callus is transformed into a rigid calcified tissue called woven bone. This bone callus forms at the periphery of the fracture site where the strain on the bone is lowest.

The remodeling stage starts when the fracture has united with the woven bone. Lamellar bone slowly replaces the woven bone the osteonal remodeling. This stage is the longest in that it can last several months to years.

Each phase has distinct characteristics; however, they have a seamless transition from one phase to the other.[8-10] Primary fracture healing and secondary fracture healing undergo different lengths of phases of bone healing as well, in that hard and soft callus formation is minimal in primary fracture healing.

As already mentioned, primary healing is achieved by absolute stability by means of interfragmentary compression. In an arthrodesis, 2 or more joint surfaces are denuded of cartilage, and the opposing subchondral bone ends are stabilized and compacted so the remaining bone can be maintained in permanent apposition. Histologically, the healing of bone undergoing primary healing requires no movement across the bone ends so the initial hematoma, formed during the stages of bone healing, is resorbed rather quickly and transformed into repair tissue. Next the Haversian system begins to repair the intricate network of systems that were once in the bone. The Haversian system is reformed by the use of an osteon, which carries at its tip a cluster of osteoclasts acting as drills that tunnel into the dead bone. After the dead bone has been resorbed, osteoblasts from behind the tip create new bone and a connection to the capillaries within the canal.

BIOMECHANICAL CONSIDERATIONS

Surgical intervention of the foot and ankle cannot be performed without careful evaluation of the biomechanical forces acting on the foot and ankle. Excessive pronation beyond the initial 25% of the stance phase of gait can be considered pathologic.[11] Pronation involves adduction and plantarflexion of the talus along with calcaneal eversion. The instability of the talocalcaneal joint causes midtarsal joint unlocking, which causes pathologic changes both distally and proximally.[12] Unlocking of the midtarsal joint during the propulsive phase of gait can lead to a hypermobile first ray,[13] which in turn can lead to a hallux rigidus.[14] Pronation can cause posterior tibial tendon dysfunction, which can lead to an associated abduction of the forefoot relative to the rearfoot.[15] Ankle joint range of motion lies primarily in the sagittal plane, with some motion occurring in the transverse plane.[16] Subtalar acts as a torque converter between the leg and the foot, translating external/internal rotational forces in the leg to pronatory/supinatory forces in the foot. When this conversion of forces fails to reach equilibrium, pain sets in.

PRINCIPLES AND INDICATIONS FOR ARTHRODESIS OF THE FOOT AND ANKLE

The principles of arthrodesis require a simple yet precise set of requirements that must be performed for successful fusion to occur. These principles include (1) complete removal of the articular cartilage and fibrous tissue from the joint to expose raw bone, (2) accurate and continuously maintained apposition of the prepared surfaces, (3) careful evaluation of angular relationships to the fused joint and augmentation using bone grafting procedures, and (4) undisturbed maintenance of the fusion site until fusion is complete.[17] A regional overview of the indications for arthrodesis of the foot and ankle is the focus of this section.

Hallux Interphalangeal Joint Fusion

Correction of a fixed deformity and instability of the hallux after trauma are indications for the arthrodesis of the hallux interphalangeal joint. This type of arthrodesis is commonly performed with a transfer of the extensor hallucis longus tendon, as in a Jones-type arthrodesis procedure. Under normal biomechanical circumstances there is little dorsiflexion of the hallux interphalangeal joint. Instability of the hallux interphalangeal joint can cause this dorsiflexion, which results in a decrease of passive plantarflexion of the of the hallux interphalangeal joint. This dorsal instability can become a damaging condition, and can cause concomitant limited dorsiflexion of the hallux metatarsophalangeal joint.[18]

Further indications for the hallux interphalangeal joint fusion include correction of a fixed deformity when associated with a neuromuscular condition, causing diffuse claw-toe deformity as in the case of a hereditary sensory motor neuropathy like Charcot-Marie-Tooth disease. Arthrodesis of the hallux interphalangeal joint is performed in conjunction with an extensor hallucis longus tendon lengthening or transfer of the extensor hallucis longus to the first metatarsal. Arthrodesis of the hallux interphalangeal joint is indicated for claw-toe deformity that is rigid or flexible because of a failed previous resection of the base of the proximal phalanx and with an intact metatarsophalangeal joint. A resection arthroplasty of the hallux (Keller procedure) that has failed is another indication for hallux interphalangeal joint correction. Correction can be achieved by arthrodesing either just the hallux interphalangeal joint or the metatarsophalangeal joint, or both.[19] Decision to arthrodese one or more joints is based on the presence of a fixed contracture and the degree of the deformity. The presence of a cock-up deformity of hallux with a flexible hallux interphalangeal joint in the setting of metatarsophalangeal dorsal instability calls for hallux interphalangeal joint arthrodesis.

Arthrodesis of the Hallux Metatarsophalangeal Joint

A fusion of the hallux metatarsophalangeal (MTP) joint can be performed in the setting of hallux rigidus, hallux varus, hallux valgus, arthridites of the MTP joint such as Gouty arthritis, and as a salvage procedure for failed hallux valgus correction.[20] The decision to perform an arthrodesis of the hallux MTP joint should be considered only as an alternative to other corrective procedures of the hallux MTP joint.

The uniqueness of the hallux MTP joint in surgical arthrodesis is evident in the anatomy of the joint itself, specifically, the sesamoids. Articulating with the plantar surface of the first metatarsal head and contained within the tendons of the flexor hallucis brevis (FHB), the sesamoids help to lengthen the lever arm of the FHB so that the muscular forces can act more efficiently on the hallux MTP joint. After an arthrodesis procedure of the hallux MTP joint the sesamoids typically retract, due to the surgical release of the flexor brevis attachment. However, this is not the case when arthrodesis is recommended for patients with arthrosis in and around the hallux MTP joint. In these patients the sesamoids become embedded into the surrounding soft-tissue structures, and the position will not change. Dissection and release of the attachments to the sesamoids will alleviate this problem.

As already mentioned, the purpose of the sesamoids is to help lengthen the moment arm of the FHB; however; performing a hallux MTP joint arthrodesis improves the lever arm of the hallux itself, resulting in increased load-bearing function of the hallux and first metatarsal.[21] Furthermore, the weight-bearing effect of the hallux MTP joint after arthrodesis was analyzed using optical pedobarographs, which showed an improved function of the hallux and increased weight bearing of the medial column.[22]

Arthrodesis of the Tarsometatarsal and Midtarsal Joints

The tarsometatarsal articulation of the foot consists of the medial, middle, and lateral columns. The medial column consists of the medial cuneiform and the first metatarsal, the middle column is the middle and lateral cuneiforms and the second and third metatarsals, and the lateral column is the fourth and fifth metatarsals and the cuboid.[23] Closed reduction after a fracture or dislocation of the tarsometatarsal joints causes shortening of the medial column with dorsiflexion, pronation of the midfoot, and abduction of the forefoot. Compensatory changes occur to the soft-tissue structures as well, including contracture of the extensor hallucis longus and extensor hallucis brevis, and attenuation of the posterior tibial, abductor hallucis, and peroneal tendons, especially the peroneus brevis. These compensatory changes lead to an increase in posttraumatic arthritis in these patients. The treatment goal for these patients must be to provide a stable and anatomic reduction regardless of the mechanism, because of the potential for increased morbidity in these patients.[24] Surgical treatment with rigid internal or external fixation should be the main goal in patients with these types of injuries. Proper diagnosis of these injuries is paramount to any treatment protocol. It is the nature of medicine to classify fractures into systems. Although classification schemes are appropriate for the academic setting, they lead to misdiagnosis and subsequently mistreatment of the underlying cause if a cookie-cutter approach is taken to fractures. Each patient must be treated differently. Patients with high-energy trauma to the foot and ankle joints can have articular cartilage that is fractured and frayed or subchondral bone that has been crushed. Imaging studies such as radiographs help to determine fractures and some articular damage that are overt in nature. A computed tomography scan with a 3-dimensional reconstruction would best benefit the preoperative considerations for surgically managing a patient with a tarsometatarsal and midtarsal joint arthrodesis procedure.

Arthrodesis of the Hindfoot

Hindfoot arthrodesis must be approached as a salvage operation when other techniques such as tendon transfers or osteotomies have failed. Flexible joints should not undergo hindfoot arthrodesis. Rigid hindfoot joints in which the deformity is a progressive one should be the main indication for arthrodesis of the hindfoot joints. These considerations for hindfoot arthrodesis are necessary because fusions change the normal biomechanics of the joint and, by definition, restrict motion at the joint, while arthrodesis procedures place increased stress on the proximal and distal joints. After triple arthrodesis, patients have 16% restriction of plantarflexion and 13% restriction of dorsiflexion.[25] In patients who undergo triple arthrodesis there is a 50% reduction of ankle joint range of motion in older individuals.[26,27]

Subtalar joint arthrodesis is a reliable procedure to stabilize a degenerative hindfoot. The procedure is indicated for posttraumatic, rheumatoid, or degenerative arthritis localized at the talocalcaneal joint, neuromuscular disorders, and hindfoot valgus deformities associated with posterior tibial tendon dysfunction. Subtalar joint arthrodesis can also be indicated in older patients who have symptomatic talocalcaneal coalitions, which do not present with significant arthritis in the transverse tarsal joints. Studies reporting radiographic degenerative changes occurring after isolated subtalar joint arthrodesis in the talonavicular and calcaneocuboid joints have been rarely clinically significant.[28–31] Patients undergoing triple arthrodesis can develop clinically significant degenerative arthritis of the midfoot and ankle.[32–34] Isolated subtalar arthrodesis is a technically less demanding procedure and, due to its joint preservation qualities, is the mainstay of arthrodesis for isolated subtalar joint arthritis.

Double arthrodesis involves fusion of the calcaneocuboid and talonavicular joints. Indications for this procedure are a severe valgus deformity of the hindfoot and degenerative joint disease of the transverse tarsal joints.[35,36] Patients presenting with a stage 4 posterior tibial tendon dysfunction or rupture of the tendon, and patients with hindfoot muscle paralysis can benefit from a double arthrodesis.

Triple arthrodesis involves the fusion of the calcaneocuboid, talocalcaneal, and talonavicular joints. Historically this procedure was first used to manage paralytic deformities of the foot and ankle in children with poliomyelitis, Charcot-Marie-Tooth disease, and cerebral palsy.[37] At present, the triple arthrodesis procedure is indicated for patients with severe pes planovalgus deformity, rheumatoid arthritis, osteoarthritis, salvage procedure for failed calcaneal fracture repair, or diabetic neuroarthropathy.[38–41] Goals of this surgery include relief of a painful foot, correction of the deformity, and the use of a plantigrade foot.

Arthrodesis of the Ankle

Ankle arthrodesis has been indicated in situations of a similar nature to those for triple arthrodesis. It has been used for failed total ankle arthroplasty, neuroarthropathy, revisional ankle arthrodesis, posttraumatic and primary arthrosis, osteoarthritis, and rheumatoid arthritis.[36,42–47] Following basic principles of arthrodesis, Charnley advocated that a compression type of arthrodesis be performed at the ankle. Ankle implants are becoming increasingly popular as more and more devices are put on the market. Salvage procedures of infected or defective total ankle replacements are restricted mainly to ankle arthrodesis, due to insufficient availability of revision implants.[48] In revisional ankle replacement arthrodesis, the surgeon is confronted with extensive bone loss, fracture and erosion of the malleoli, a vulnerable soft tissue envelope, and deficient talar contact areas. Indications for ankle revisional arthrodesis are failure of the prosthesis, loose ankle total replacement, severe ankle destruction and axial deviation in rheumatoid patients, and severe osteoarthritis in subtalar joint and ankle joint. The use of bone graft and secure fixation can assist the surgeon in arthrodesis of the ankle with a failed implant. This procedure avoids a limb length discrepancy, allows correction of hindfoot deformity in retrograde nail arthrodesis, and reduces disturbed wound healing by resection of the distal fibula, while no external fixation is required. If infection is present, two-stage revisional surgery is typically performed.[48]

REFERENCES

1. Gray H, Standring S, Ellis H, et al. Gray's anatomy: the anatomical basis of clinical practice. 39th edition. Edinburgh, New York: Elsevier Churchill Livingstone; 2005.
2. Valmassy R. Clinical biomechanics of the lower extremities. St Louis (MO): Mosby; 1996.
3. Hall BK. Cartilage. New York: Academic Press; 1983.

4. Schoutens A. Bone circulation and vascularization in normal and pathological conditions. New York: Plenum Press; 1993.
5. Turner CH, Wang T, Burr DB. Shear strength and fatigue properties of human cortical bone determined from pure shear tests. Calcif Tissue Int 2001;69(6):373–8.
6. Reilly DT, Burstein AH. The elastic and ultimate properties of compact bone tissue. J Biomech 1975;8(6):393–405.
7. Brookes M, Revell WJ. Blood supply of bone: scientific aspects. Rev. and updated. London, New York: Springer; 1998.
8. Peters A, Schell H, Bail HJ, et al. Standard bone healing stages occur during delayed bone healing, albeit with a different temporal onset and spatial distribution of callus tissues. Histol Histopathol 2010;25(9):1149–62.
9. Gheduzzi S, Dodd SP, Miles AW, et al. Numerical and experimental simulation of the effect of long bone fracture healing stages on ultrasound transmission across an idealized fracture. J Acoust Soc Am 2009;126(2):887–94.
10. Dodd SP, Miles AW, Gheduzzi S, et al. Modelling the effects of different fracture geometries and healing stages on ultrasound signal loss across a long bone fracture. Comput Methods Biomech Biomed Engin 2007;10(5):371–5.
11. Sgarlato T. Tendon Achilles lengthening and its effect on foot disorders. J Am Podiatry Assoc 1975;65:849.
12. Hicks J. The mechanics of the foot I. The joints. J Anat 1976;88:345–57.
13. Cornwall MW, McPoil TG, Fischco WD, et al. The influence of first ray mobility on forefoot plantar pressure and hindfoot kinematics during walking. Foot Ankle Int 2006;27(7):539–47.
14. Root ML, Orien W, Weed JH. Clinical biomechanics: normal and abnormal function of the foot, vol. 2. Los Angeles (CA): Clinical Biomechanics Corp; 1977.
15. Jahss MH. Disorders of the foot and ankle: medical and surgical management. Philadelphia: WB Saunders; 1991.
16. Inman VT, Ralston HJ, Todd F, et al. Human walking. Baltimore (MD): Williams & Wilkins; 1981.
17. Glissan DJ. The indications for inducting fusion at the ankle joint by operation, with description of two successful techniques. Aust N Z J Surg 1949;19:64–71.
18. Aas M, Johnsen TM, Finsen V. Arthrodesis of the first metatarsophalangeal joint for hallux rigidus–optimal position of fusion. Foot (Edinb) 2008;18(3):131–5.
19. Wu KK. First metatarsophalangeal fusion in the salvage of failed hallux abducto valgus operations. The Journal of foot and ankle surgery: official publication of the American College of Foot and Ankle Surgeons 1994;33(4):383–95.
20. Leaseburg JT, DeOrio JK, Shapiro SA. Radiographic correlation of hallux MP fusion position and plate angle. Foot Ankle Int 2009;30(9):873–6.
21. Henry AP, Waugh W, Wood H. The use of footprints in assessing the results of operations for hallux valgus: a comparison of Keller's operation and arthrodesis. J Bone Joint Surg Br 1975;57:478.
22. Beauchamp C, Kirby T, Rudge SR, et al. Fusion of the first metatarsophalangeal joint in forefoot arthroplasty. Clin Orthop 1984;190:249.
23. Mann RA, Prieskorn D, Sobel M. Mid-tarsal and tarsometatarsal arthrodesis for primary degenerative osteoarthrosis or osteoarthrosis after trauma. J Bone Joint Surg Am 1996;78:1376.
24. Komenda GA, Myerson MS, Biddinger KR. Results of arthrodesis of the tarsometatarsal joints after traumatic injury. J Bone Joint Surg Am 1996;78(11):1665–76.
25. Fisher J. New ways to heal fractures enter the market, in the works. Orthop Today 1996;16(1):24–6.

26. Graves SC, Mann R, Graves KO. Triple arthrodesis in older adults. J Bone Joint Surg Am 1993;75:355–62.
27. Sc G. Triple arthrodesis in adults: indications, technique, and results. Operat Tech Orthop 1992;2:151–6.
28. Diezi C, Favre P, Vienne P. Primary isolated subtalar arthrodesis: outcome after 2 to 5 years followup. Foot Ankle Int 2008;29(12):1195–202.
29. Myerson M, Quill GE Jr. Late complications of fractures of the calcaneus. J Bone Joint Surg Am 1993;75(3):331–41.
30. Kile TA, Donnelly RE, Gehrke JC, et al. Tibiotalocalcaneal arthrodesis with an intramedullary device. Foot Ankle Int 1994;15(12):669–73.
31. Hoke M. An operation for stabilizing paralytic feet. Am J Orthop Surg 1921;3:4949.
32. Grant WP, Garcia-Lavin S, Sabo R. Beaming the columns for Charcot diabetic foot reconstruction: a retrospective analysis. J Foot Ankle Surg 2011;50(2):182–9.
33. DeCarbo WT, Berlet GC, Hyer CF, et al. Single-screw fixation for subtalar joint fusion does not increase nonunion rate. Foot Ankle Spec 2010;3(4):164–6.
34. Tuijthof GJ, Beimers L, Kerkhoffs GM, et al. Overview of subtalar arthrodesis techniques: options, pitfalls and solutions. Foot Ankle Surg 2010;16(3):107–16.
35. Mann RA, Beaman DN. Double arthrodesis in the adult. Clin Orthop Relat Res 1999;365:74–80.
36. Beischer AD, Brodsky JW, Pollo FE, et al. Functional outcome and gait analysis after triple or double arthrodesis. Foot Ankle Int 1999;20(9):545–53.
37. Ryerson EW. Arthrodesing operations on the feet: Edwin W. Ryerson MD (1872-1961). The 1st president of the AAOS 1932. Clin Orthop Relat Res 2008;466(1):5–14.
38. Napiontek M, Pietrzak K. Triple arthrodesis of the foot after calcaneal fractures. Twelve patients treated using K wires stabilization. Foot Ankle Surg 2011;17(3):128–30.
39. Brink DS, Eickmeier KM, Levitsky DR, et al. Subtalar and talonavicular joint dislocation as a presentation of diabetic neuropathic arthropathy with salvage by triple arthrodesis. J Foot Ankle Surg 1994;33(6):583–9.
40. Pakarinen TK, Laine HJ, Honkonen SE, et al. Charcot arthropathy of the diabetic foot. Current concepts and review of 36 cases. Scand J Surg 2002;91(2):195–201.
41. Myerson MS, Edwards WH. Management of neuropathic fractures in the foot and ankle. J Am Acad Orthop Surg 1999;7(1):8–18.
42. Wukich DK, Shen JY, Ramirez CP, et al. Retrograde ankle arthrodesis using an intramedullary nail: a comparison of patients with and without diabetes mellitus. J Foot Ankle Surg 2011;50(3):299–306.
43. Tulner S, Klinkenbijl M, Albers G. Revision arthrodesis of the ankle: a 4 cannulated screw compression fixation technique. Acta Orthop 2011;82(2):250–2.
44. Charnley J. Compression arthrodesis of the ankle and shoulder. J Bone Joint Surg Br 1951;33B(2):180–91.
45. Krause FG, Windolf M, Bora B, et al. Impact of complications in total ankle replacement and ankle arthrodesis analyzed with a validated outcome measurement. J Bone Joint Surg Am 2011;93(9):830–9.
46. Clare MP, Sanders RW. The anatomic compression arthrodesis technique with anterior plate augmentation for ankle arthrodesis. Foot Ankle Clin 2011;16(1):91–101.
47. Torudom Y. The results of ankle arthrodesis with screws for end stage ankle arthrosis. J Med Assoc Thai 2010;93(Suppl 2):S50–4.
48. Schill S. Ankle arthrodesis with interposition graft as a salvage procedure after failed total ankle replacement. Oper Orthop Traumatol 2007;19(5–6):547–60 [in German].

Complications of Arthrodesis and Nonunion

Jeffrey Martone, DPM[a,b,c,d,*], Laura Vander Poel, DPM[e],
Nadia Levy, DPM[e]

KEYWORDS

- Nonunion • Fusion • Bone healing • Pseudoarthrosis
- Internal fixation

Arthrodesis has long been used as a viable surgical option by many foot and ankle surgeons. Joint fusions have historically been viewed as a good choice for those patients whose particular foot and ankle pathology requires a definitive, stabilizing procedure.[1] Some of the more common conditions addressed by fusion include trauma, arthritis, and congenital or developmental malalignment syndromes.[1] Arthrodesis is often an ideal solution for a painful or degenerated joint; unfortunately, the procedure does not come without a set of potential complications that can prove to be challenging.

Complications of joint fusions can include those applicable to any surgery such as bone and/or soft-tissue infection, wound dehiscence, and failure of fixation. Other complications are specific to fusion procedures and would include malalignment, proximal or distal joint deterioration, and delayed union or nonunion.[1] The latter negative outcomes can occur from medical comorbidities, patient noncompliance, or inappropriate fixation.

This article attempts to address many of these complications including techniques for evaluation, accurate diagnosis, and current treatment options. Special attention is

The authors have nothing to disclose.
[a] Temple School of Medicine, School of Podiatric Medicine, 148 North 8th Street, Philadelphia, PA 19107-2418, USA
[b] Barry University, School of Podiatric Medicine, 11300 Northeast 2nd Avenue, Miami Shores, FL 33161-6695, USA
[c] Dr William M. Scholl School of Podiatric Medicine, Rosalind Franklin University, 3333 Green Bay Road, North Chicago, IL 60064-3095, USA
[d] Private Practice, Department of Surgery, Saint Francis Hospital and Medical Center, East Hartford, CT 06108, USA
[e] Department of Surgery, Saint Francis Hospital and Medical Center, 114 Woodland Street, Hartford, CT 06105, USA
* Corresponding author. Private Practice, Department of Surgery, Saint Francis Hospital and Medical Center, East Hartford, CT 06108.
E-mail address: doctormartone@yahoo.com

Clin Podiatr Med Surg 29 (2012) 11–18
doi:10.1016/j.cpm.2011.09.002
0891-8422/12/$ – see front matter © 2012 Elsevier Inc. All rights reserved.

paid to the subject of nonunion, as it is one of the most common and difficult adverse outcomes of arthrodesis procedures.

PRINCIPLES OF ARTHRODESIS AND BONE HEALING

As with any surgical condition, the decision-making process is paramount to the success of the case. The selection of a joint fusion procedure is made with the knowledge that the affected joint will no longer have its intended function and motion.[1,2] In most cases this is a beneficial consequence because the joint structure has already lost its motion or structural integrity through injury or degeneration, leaving the patient with pain and loss of function. Arthrodesis can eliminate patient's pain while providing stability of the previously malfunctioning or nonfunctioning joint.[1,2] However, there are examples when the surgeon may opt to fuse a joint prophylactically to avoid future problems; such is the case following severe fractures involving a joint. It is important to weigh the advantages against the disadvantages before undertaking this kind of preemptive fusion.

Arthrodesis requires diligent anatomic dissection, complete articular cartilage resection, accurate realignment, and stable fixation. These concepts are critical for primary bone healing to take place.[2]

Bone healing can be separated into primary or secondary healing.[3,4] Primary bone healing occurs with rigid stabilization enhanced by compression, and preservation of vascularity. It occurs with either contact or gap healing, where the gap is less than 2 mm.[3–5] This type of bone healing involves Haversian remodeling, where cutting cones phagocytose osteoids and lay down new lamellar bone. Secondary bone healing can also lead to successful arthrodesis, but is considered less desirable because there is micromotion and an extra bone callus formation phase.[3,4] The less the stability and callus formation, the more delay there will be for complete bone healing.

CAUSES OF COMPLICATION AND NONUNION

There are several types of complications of arthrodesis. For the purpose of this discussion they are separated into technical and biologic complications.[6–8]

Technical complications relate more to the surgeon and include poor surgical selection, execution of procedure, or inadequate fixation and/or stabilization (**Fig. 1**). Patient noncompliance can play a large role in the problems, due to fixation and stability. These complications are often a result of ill-prepared surgery and are often avoidable.[2]

Arthrodesis procedures are among the most technically challenging and demanding procedures for the foot and ankle surgeon. Adequate training and experience is paramount to the success of the procedure. Dissection of the fusion site that fails to

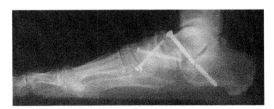

Fig. 1. Example of fixation failure; broken hardware.

preserve the neurovascular supply will undoubtedly result in a decreased healing capacity.[7,8] In some cases, disruption of vascular supply can lead to avascular necrosis, and nerve damage can also lead to a condition called complex regional pain syndrome.

Even with completed fusion, poor alignment will cause problems with stability, gait, shoe fit, and patient function.[8] Finally, inadequate fixation can allow motion across the arthrodesis site and lead to delayed union or nonunion, and possibly displacement of reduction (**Fig. 2**).[6–8]

Biologic complications are those that arise from physiologic sources, making them difficult to fully control or avoid. The most prevalent biologic complication is a surgical infection. Surgical infections are not common; however, the likelihood can increase in patients with certain medical comorbidities. Any condition that may cause the patient a decrease in immune response can increase the patient's chance of a surgical infection. These conditions include, but are not limited to, diabetes mellitus, peripheral vascular compromise, immunosuppression, and tobacco use.[9,10] Numerous studies have shown that any one of these conditions will significantly affect healing. Fortunately, the use of perioperative antibiotics is almost universally applicable in fusion cases, and will inevitably minimize the risk. Proper surgical dissection and periosteal and soft-tissue closure must be performed to ensure

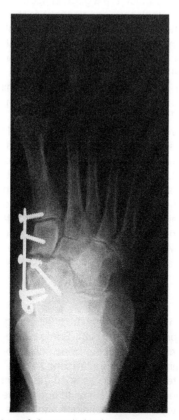

Fig. 2. Example of a nonunion of the medial column.

adequate blood supply. Most important is the concept of patient selection.[1–3,7,8] A patient who has significant or multiple comorbidities may not be a candidate for any type of surgical arthrodesis. Other methods for treatment must be used if the risk of complication is too great.

Mention must be made here of patient noncompliance. Even with a perfect operative technique, a patient who does not faithfully participate in his or her own care will be at great risk for complications. It is in these most difficult cases that the surgeon must accept the limits of training, skill, and medical technology, and implement other more predictable and safe treatment options.

CLASSIFICATION AND DIAGNOSIS OF NONUNION

Nonunions are one of the most daunting complications of arthrodesis procedures, and deserve special mention. By definition, a delayed union is when a reasonable period of time elapses without any indication of arthrodesis. A nonunion is defined as failure to achieve union after approximately 9 months of treatment time. However, this does not imply that one must wait 9 months before intervention. The most important determinant for a nonunion is its vascular supply.[6–8] The pattern and distribution of the vessels at a fusion site will determine what treatment options are available to achieve fusion.

A hypervascular nonunion has a good healing potential, due to its proliferation of vessels at the fusion site.[1,6–8] There are subclasses of hypervascular nonunion based on their radiographic patterns, which are a good indicator of bone activity and healing potential. The radiographic subclasses are elephant-foot pattern, horse-hoof pattern, and oligotrophic pattern. All of these patterns are a type of pseudoarthrosis.[6–8]

The elephant-foot pattern has a wide pattern of bone callus formation that extends well beyond the nonunion site.[1,7,8] The horse-hoof pattern has less callus but still extends beyond the normal bone diameter. These patterns are most often associated with motion at the fusion site.[1,7,8] Oligotrophic is the third type of hypervascular nonunion, in which there is much less callus formation implying less vascularity and a low potential for healing.[1,7,8]

Avascular nonunions have inadequate blood supply and little osteogenic potential. These nonunions are classified into comminuted, torsion wedge, defect/void, and atrophic patterns.[1,7,8] The comminuted and torsion wedge have incomplete and partial healing of fragments, which has no application in arthrodesis nonunion. Defect nonunion can apply when aggressive joint resection and inadequate grafting lead to a void between bones and poor bone bridging.[1,7,8] An atrophic nonunion is one that has formed over a significant period of time during which the bones have undergone breakdown and resorption. There is often devitalized bone present that requires adequate resection to fully heal. This nonunion will have no osseous integrity and will often lead to a structural collapse.[6]

DIAGNOSING NONUNION

Diagnosing a delayed union or nonunion can be challenging, but is the most important step in establishing a proper treatment plan. Some of the generally accepted diagnostic tools include plain film radiography, bone scan, computed tomography (CT), magnetic resonance imaging (MRI), and ultrasonography.[1,7,8] As with most medical conditions, none of these techniques are as accurate or important as the physician's clinical evaluation. A high index of suspicion and aggressive treatment are paramount to successful outcomes. Any imaging technique should be thought of as a confirmatory measure or a helpful aid for further treatment planning.

The progress of bone healing is readily viewable on plain film radiographs. Several of the phases of bone healing are typically visible on the radiographs over the typical 6-week bone-healing time.[1,7,8] The inflammatory phase progresses to the soft callus phase, then on to hard callus, and finally remodeling. If stable fixation is used these phases are subtle[6,7]; they may include blurring of the fusion site interface that progresses to trabecular bone seen crossing the fusion site.[1,7,8] The formation of external callus can indicate secondary healing; however, as mentioned previously, this does not always result in nonunion. The formation of external callus with persistent gapping at the arthrodesis site combined with lucency around fixation are all common indicators seen in early nonunion.[1,7,8]

When plain radiographs fail to confirm nonunion and a high clinical suspicion is present, other modalities may be used. A 3-phase technetium bone scan can be useful for evaluating activity of bone.[6–8] Bone scans are highly sensitive and can show patterns of bone healing at fracture and fusion ends, and even show vascular ingrowth patterns for graft material.[1,7,8]

CT and MRI modalities can differentiate the various tissue stages present at the site of fusion healing. MRI can differentiate between soft and hard callus formation, soft-tissue interposition and, when combined with the use of contrast, the vascularity of these different tissues.[1,6–8] For these reasons, it is the most useful imaging technique for planning revisional surgery. Unfortunately, the use of MRI can be restricted in certain cases because of artifact from metallic fixation, but a skilled technician can often alter test parameters to evaluate areas of suspected pathology.

A note of caution must be made here regarding the use of time as an indicator for diagnosing nonunion. Although it is widely used as a determinant for coverage of certain nonunion treatment options, it is nonscientific and highly unreliable.[6] The phases of bone healing are well known, but every patient and every case will heal within their own unique time frame. A nonunion by definition is a fusion or fracture that has not adequately healed,[1] which may occur early or late in the postoperative period, and should be treated at the time it is diagnosed, not at an arbitrary point in time.

TREATMENT

Early and aggressive treatment of any arthrodesis complication is essential for good clinical outcomes. Once an accurate diagnosis is made, treatment options will become apparent. Treatment can be separated into nonsurgical and surgical.

Nonsurgical treatments of fusion complications use modalities that rely on the assumption that the patient has the physiologic capacity to heal.[1] If the anatomic reduction and arthrodesis position are stable and the patient shows evidence of good bone-healing potential, then nonsurgical methods are appropriate.

Nonsurgical Treatment

Immobilization is critical for adequate bone healing. Maintaining correction and position and preventing motion will allow for boney ingrowth across the proposed fusion site and bone healing to occur.[1,8] Immobilization may be achieved by a plaster or fiberglass cast. The compliant patient can achieve the same result using a removable type of cast, which may provide the additional convenience of bathing, wound care, and pin-site maintenance when needed.[1,7,8] In addition to immobilization, external bone stimulation is a proven adjunct to bone healing. Types of bone stimulators are differentiated by their technologies; ultrasound, electrical, and magnetic.[11–15]

Ultrasound-based bone stimulation uses pulsed, low-intensity ultrasound to stimulate the aggregation and production of certain proteins useful for bone healing,[11,12] accomplished through a transducer with a conductive coupling gel placed on the skin over the nonunion or fracture site.

Electrical stimulation has 3 distinct technologies. A pulsed electromagnetic field uses a low-energy direct current that is converted into a pulsed current via an electrical coil placed over the failed arthrodesis fusion or fracture nonunion site.[11] An example of this technology is used in the EBI Bone Healing System (**Fig. 3**).

Capacitative coupling delivers a constant current of low-intensity energy via electrode pads placed on the skin over the treatment site.[11] This technology is used in the OrthoPak and SpinalPak bone stimulators (**Fig. 4**).

Finally, combined magnetic field (CMF) combines a dynamic and static magnetic field to create an even electric current to the nonunion or fracture site through an external coil. The DonJoy OL-1000 uses CMF technology.[11–16]

While each of these technologies are slightly different, they are all thought to upregulate several osteoinductive growth factors including bone morphogenic protein (BMP), an essential protein seen in all bone healing.[11,13] In addition, success rates vary but each manufacturer has demonstrated healing rates above 80%, making external bone stimulation a viable treatment option. The greatest difference between the various bone stimulators is in their respective treatment parameters for time of application, and depth of tissue penetration.[11–16]

Surgical Treatment

Surgical measures to address a failed fusion must be used when immobilization, bone stimulation, and other conservative measures have failed. Surgery is also mandated if the position of a completed fusion is not mechanically sound, or if fixation has failed. It

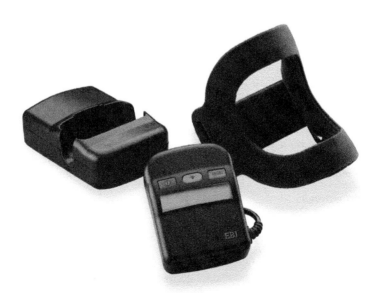

Fig. 3. EBI Bone Healing System. (*Courtesy of* Biomet Spine & Bone Healing Technologies, Parsippany, NJ; with permission.)

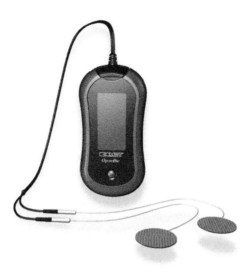

Fig. 4. OrthoPak 2 Bone Growth Stimulator. (*Courtesy of* Biomet Spine & Bone Healing Technologies, Parsippany, NJ; with permission.)

is necessary, of course, to determine the cause of failure. Often biological causes cannot be addressed by surgery.

Technical complications are more amenable to surgical options. Replacing or augmenting surgical fixation may provide additional stability to achieve fusion. The presence of a fibrous or cartilaginous pseudoarthrosis is an absolute surgical indicator.[2,7,8] Resection of the nonviable pseudoarthrosis and the addition of bone or platelet-rich graft materials are critical to introduce growth factors to an area of poor healing potential and to allow boney ingrowth.[17–19] The most difficult surgical correction involves the completed arthrodesis in poor mechanical position.[2] This method is technically difficult for the surgeon, who must now destroy a healed procedure, then realign and refixate the limb. It is arguably more difficult for the patient, who must incur another surgical procedure with all the inherent risks as well as a second recovery period.[1,2,7,8]

SUMMARY

Arthrodesis is a useful but technically demanding procedure for the foot and ankle surgeon. As such, it is a procedure with many potential complications. Choosing the correct patient and procedure, types of fixation, dissection technique, proper positioning, and appropriate convalescence and therapy are all paramount to the success of the surgical procedure. When a complication occurs, understanding the type and etiology of the complication is the most important first step toward treatment. By using available technology to make an accurate diagnosis and by applying treatment early and aggressively, good clinical outcomes and high patient satisfaction are likely.

REFERENCES

1. Banks AS, Downey MS, Martin DE, et al. McGlamry's comprehensive textbook of foot and ankle surgery, volume one and two. 3rd edition. Chapter 37: Rearfoot

arthrodesis and Chapter 64: Augmentation of bone growth and healing, Philadelphia, 2001.
2. Chang T. Masters techniques in podiatric surgery. The Foot and Ankle, 2004.
3. Rahn BA, Gallinaro P, Baltensperger A, et al. Primary Bone healing. J Bone and Joint Surgery 1971;53:783–6.
4. McKibbon B. The biology of fracture healing in long bones. J Bone and Joint Surgery 1978;60B:150.
5. Chalmers J, Gray DH, Rush J. Observations on the induction of bone in soft tissues. J Bone and Joint Surgery 1975;57:36.
6. Oloff L, Jacobs A. Fracture nonunion. In: Scurran B, editor. Clinics in Podiatry, vol 2. Philadelphia (PA): WB Saunders; 1985.
7. Mayer PJ, Evarts CM. Nonunion, delayed union, malunion and avascular necrosis. In: Epps CH Jr, editor. Complications in orthopedic surgery, vol 1. 2nd edition. Philadelphia: JB Lippincott; 1986.
8. Taylor JC. Delayed union and nonunion in fractures. In: Crenshaw A, editor. Campbell's Operative Orthopedics, vol 2. 8th edition. St. Louis: CV Mosby; 1992.
9. Cobb TK, Gabrielson TA, Campbell DC III, et al. Cigarette smoking and nonunion after ankle arthrodesis. Foot and Ankle Int 1995;15:64.
10. Siverstein P. Smoking and wound healing. Am J Med 1992;93:22.
11. Bassett CAL, Mitchell SN, Gasten S. Treatment of ununited tibial diaphyseal fracture with pulsing electromagnetic field. J Bone and Joint Surgery 1981;63A:511.
12. Brighton CT. Biophysics of fracture healing. In: Heppenstall RB, editor. Fracture treatment and healing. Philadelphia: WB Saunders; 1980.
13. Brighton CT. The treatment of nonunions with electricity. J Bone and Joint Surgery 1981;21P:63A.
14. BioMet. Bone growth stimulators. Biomet, Inc; 2011. Available at: http://www.biomet.com/trauma/products.cfm?pdid=4&majcid=47. Accessed July 30, 2011.
15. CMF bone growth stimulation. DJO, LLC; 2011. Available at: http://apps.djoglobal.com/bonestim/products/. Accessed July 30, 2011.
16. Smith&Nephew. Exogen bone healing system. Smith&Nephew; 2011. Available at: http://global.smith-nephew.com/us/patients/EXOGEN_BONE_HEALING_SYS_14437.htm?Nav=false?status=show. Accessed July 30, 2011.
17. Nicholl EA. Treatment of gaps in long bones by cancellous insert grafts. J bone and Joint Surgery 1956;38B:70–82.
18. Heppenstall BR. The present role of bone graft surgery in treating nonunion. Orthopedic Clinics North America 1984;15:113.
19. Mahan KT. Bone graft materials and perioperative management. In: Camasta CA, editor. Reconstructive Surgery of the Foot and Leg: update '95. Tucker (GA): Podiatry Institute; 1995.

Master Techniques in Digital Arthrodesis

Albert M. D'Angelantonio, BSME, DPM[a,b,]*,
Kaitlin A. Nelson-Rinaldi, DPM[a], Jade Barnard, DPM[a],
Frank Oware, DPM[a]

KEYWORDS

- Digital arthrodesis • Digital fusion
- Interphalangeal joint arthrodesis
- Interphalangeal intramedullary implant

HISTORICAL BACKGROUND

In 1910, Soule[1] first described the intentional arthrodesis of the proximal interphalangeal joint (PIPJ). Further advances have allowed for increased stability of digital arthrodesis procedures. For example, in 1931, Higgs[2] advocated fusion using a spike-and-hole method. Young[3] developed a similar peg-in-hole configuration, although he remodeled the proximal phalanx into a truncated cone shape. In 1940, Taylor[4] was credited with the first use of Kirschner wire (K-wire) intramedullary fixation in hammer toe surgery. To prevent proximal migration of the K-wire, Selig[5] further suggested that the hardware be bent at its distal margin, significantly improving the reliability of this form of fixation. More recent innovations include absorbable fixation and intramedullary digital implants.

HISTORY AND PHYSICAL EXAMINATION

Patients complaining of digital deformities may report varying degrees of symptoms. Dorsal pain may be caused by pressure from footwear, which leads to callosities, whereas pain at the distal end of the toe may be secondary to contracture and the resultant shift of pressure from the more plantar padded metatarsal heads to the toe.[6] Patients tend to report a history of digital deformity since birth or early childhood. Patients may relate that the extent of deformity has reached an end point or may note continued progression of the deformity. Patients commonly complain of difficulty fitting into shoes because of the severity of digital deformity. Usually the pain is exacerbated by pressure from footwear. Nonunion phalangeal fracture may be a cause of

[a] Podiatric Medicine and Surgery, Kennedy University Hospital, 18 East Laurel Road, Stratford, NJ 08084, USA
[b] Regional Foot and Ankle Specialists, 188 Fries Mill Road, Suite N2, Turnersville, NJ 08012, USA
* Corresponding author. Regional Foot and Ankle Specialists, 188 Fries Mill Road, Suite N2, Turnersville, NJ 08012.
E-mail address: aldangelo@comcast.net

Clin Podiatr Med Surg 29 (2012) 21–40
doi:10.1016/j.cpm.2011.10.002
0891-8422/12/$ – see front matter © 2012 Elsevier Inc. All rights reserved.

podiatric.theclinics.com

digital deformity, but this is significantly less common than congenital deformities acquired over the years.[6]

Physical examination is a vital step in preoperative planning. Evaluation should first be made regarding the patient's overall health. Poor health may eliminate the patient as a surgical candidate. A problem-focused physical examination should then be performed to evaluate the extent of digital deformity. Examination must include assessment of the circulatory status of the lower extremity. Although some surgical procedures require limited exposure, other procedures may require extensive dissection at the metatarsophalangeal joint (MPJ), at the interphalangeal joints (IPJs), or along the medial and lateral aspects of the phalanges. Whether an individual digit can withstand multiple procedures and extensive surgical exposure depends on the vascular status of the digit.

The sensory status of a foot must be evaluated as well. An impaired sensory status can indicate a systemic disease, such as diabetes, peripheral neuropathy, or lumbar disk disease. It is also important to differentiate MPJ pain from an interdigital neuroma of the adjacent intermetatarsal space.[7,8] Preoperative documentation of sensation is important because surgical dissection can diminish postoperative sensation.

A thorough biomechanical examination should also be performed. Muscle imbalance between intrinsic and extrinsic muscles of the foot usually involves multiple toes with either rigid or flexible deformities and is often associated with cavus foot with or without contracted Achilles tendon. A painful bursa may develop at the PIPJ as a result of elevated contracture of the toe. When deformity becomes rigid, the plantar fat pad is pulled distally, causing pressure callus formation in the submetatarsal area.[9] The plantar aspect of the foot should be examined for development of intractable plantar keratoses that can develop in association with contractures of the lesser toes, the result of a buckling effect of the digits. Calluses can develop pain beneath the tip of the toe or a lesser metatarsal head.[10,11] The individual digits should also be examined for callosities on the medial and lateral aspects, as well as over the IPJ and at the tip of the toe. The rigidity of the toe contractures, the position of the metatarsal, and Achilles tendon tightness should all be analyzed. Tightness of the flexor digitorum longus tendon must also be assessed. It is important to evaluate these deformities while the patient is both seated and weight bearing.

Preoperatively, it is also important to determine whether there is sufficient space to accommodate the involved toe after reduction to a normal position. The Kelikian push-up test is important in determining the appropriate procedure. Performance of the push-up test loads the metatarsals plantarly to mimic the weight-bearing position of the patient's foot. This test should be done preoperatively to determine the extent of contracture in the digit as well as intraoperatively to determine if further release of soft tissue or osteotomy is needed to relieve the contracture.[12] If a patient has a concomitant hallux valgus deformity that has diminished the interval between the first and third toes, adequate space must be obtained for the corrected lesser toe, otherwise the deformity can recur.[13] A hallux valgus repair may be necessary to obtain sufficient space between the first and third toes to realign the second toe successfully. At times, the adjacent lesser toes can drift into medial or lateral deviation, again diminishing the interval that the corrected toe should occupy. These toes may need to be corrected to afford the corrected hammer toe adequate space.

ETIOLOGY/DEFINITION

Digital deformities are generally defined based on the level of contracture. Lesser hammer toes present as a deformity primarily in the sagittal plane, with plantar flexion of the PIPJ and dorsiflexion of the MPJ. With such deformity, the middle and distal phalanges become flexed on the proximal phalanx.[14] The causes of hammer toe deformity include muscle imbalance, Charcot-Marie-Tooth disease, Friedreich ataxia, cerebral palsy, myelodysplasia, multiple sclerosis, and degenerative disk disease. Such deformities may also be associated with neuropathy secondary to diabetes mellitus and Hansen disease.[15] Progressive disease states of rheumatoid, psoriatic, and other inflammatory arthritides can also lead to hammer toe deformity.

Claw toe is a sagittal plane deformity with dorsiflexion of the MPJ and plantar flexion of the distal IPJ and PIPJ.[14] The cause of claw toe deformity is similar to that of hammer toe, including neuromuscular disease, arthritis, and metabolic disease.

Mallet toe is a sagittal plane deformity with plantar flexion of the distal IPJ.[1] The cause of mallet toe is largely unknown, although deformity has been related to recurrent pressure on the tip of the digit secondary to shoe wear. Such deformity may be associated with trauma or inflammatory arthritis or may present iatrogenically following hammer toe repair. Mallet toe is more common in women (with 84% predominance),[16] although equal frequency is observed in the second, third, and fourth toes.[10,16–21] In pediatrics, the flexor hallucis longus tendon is sometimes contracted, causing flexion at the distal IPJ. This condition is termed curly toe.[22–26]

The cause of digital deformity is closely linked to the specific time in the gait cycle when the toe becomes progressively deformed. There are 3 basic mechanisms: flexor stabilization, flexor substitution, and extensor substitution.

Flexor stabilization is the most common mechanism of deformity. This deformity occurs in a pronated foot type during the late-stance phase of gait. Common causes of flatfoot deformity include forefoot varus, equinus, calcaneal valgus, torsional abnormalities, muscle imbalances, ligament laxity, and neuromuscular disease. Early and long firing of flexor muscles occurs in an attempt to stabilize a pronated mobile forefoot. In turn, increased pull of the long flexor muscles occurs as they gain mechanical advantage over intrinsic muscles such as the interossei.[9,12,14,27] Hammer toe deformities develop when intrinsic muscles are not able to counter these deforming forces.

Extensor substitution is a swing phase condition that develops secondary to weak anterior group muscles. During this phase in the gait cycle, anterior group muscles fire to dorsiflex the foot at the ankle. Deformity develops when extensor muscles in the anterior compartment gain a mechanical advantage over intrinsic muscles such as the lumbricals. Extensor substitution can occur secondary to ankle equinus, weak lumbricals, or spasticity of the extensor digitorum longus. On physical examination, marked dorsiflexion of the MPJ is often noted, although this may straighten with weight bearing. The extensor tendons and the metatarsal heads are prominent dorsally and plantarly, respectively.[9,12,14,27] Normally the digits dorsiflex approximately 6° at the MPJs, but with extensor substitution there is more dorsiflexion of the proximal phalanges. Although the digits appear rectus on weight bearing, during swing they curl up because of extensor substitution.

Flexor substitution is a stance phase deformity occurring in a supinated foot type (Fig. 1). In this situation, the triceps surae is weak. This deficit may develop secondary to overlengthening of the Achilles tendon or may be congenital. To compensate the posterior deep muscles and the peronei, the physician must attempt to produce heel off in place of the weakened triceps. The flexors in turn gain mechanical advantage over the interossei muscles. On physical examination, a calcaneal gait and supinated high arch foot type are commonly seen with this deformity.[12]

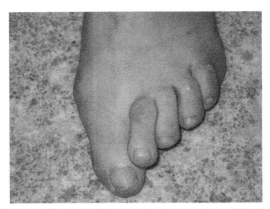

Fig. 1. Contracted cavus deformity with secondary hammering of digits.

RADIOGRAPHIC ANALYSIS

Radiographic examination is necessary to evaluate the magnitude of digital osseous deformity. During the evaluation of the patient, weight-bearing radiographs are highly recommended. These studies help in determining the extent and location of digital contractures as well as MPJ deformity and subluxation. Associated deformities such as hallux valgus or other contributing pathology such as cavus foot or metatarsus adductus should be evaluated. Radiographic evaluation may also show the presence or absence of arthritic changes, particularly those changes associated with systemic processes such as rheumatoid arthritis and inflammatory diseases. Bone scans, magnetic resonance imaging, or computed tomographic scans are rarely needed in the diagnosis of a lesser digital deformity.[6]

On an anteroposterior view, a severe hammer toe deformity can have the appearance of a gun barrel deformity (**Fig. 2**) when the proximal phalanx is seen end on. Assessment of the IPJs is difficult on the anteroposterior view. Attenuation of the metatarsophalangeal space can indicate subluxation. Overlap of the base of the proximal phalanx in relation to the metatarsal head indicates dislocation of the MPJ. Subchondral erosion, flattening of the articular surfaces, or Freiberg infraction indicate the need for further radiographic or laboratory evaluation.[12]

A lateral view may be helpful to assess the magnitude of contracture of the IPJs. Stress radiographs may also be considered to evaluate subluxability of the MPJ.[12]

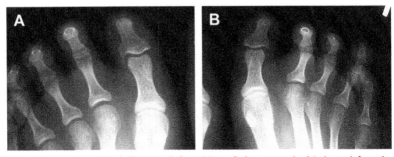

Fig. 2. (*A, B*) Interphalangeal flexion deformities of the second, third, and fourth digits, indicating a gun barrel sign.

INDICATIONS FOR FUSION

IPJ fusion should be considered in patients with the following indications:

1. Recurrence of deformity
2. Deformity of the proximal phalangeal joint in the transverse plane
3. A neuromuscular cause of the deformity
4. Inadequate flexion strength at the MPJ when stiffness of the IPJ will be acceptable to the patient
5. Requirement for a degree of predictability of surgery when the patient may not object to a stiff toe.[2,10,12,15,28–30]

Digital arthrodesis should be considered after recurrence of digital deformity. Especially in the case of failed arthroplasty, fusion may provide more favorable results. In the case of failed surgical intervention, particular attention should be directed to unaddressed deforming factors. These may include soft tissue contractures or significant deformity at the level of the MPJ.

Fusion may also be considered to address digital deformity in the transverse plane. If the MPJ is subluxated or dislocated, this deformity should be corrected simultaneously with the hammer toe correction.[15,28–30] Fusion provides more reliable realignment of multiplane digital deformities.

Digital arthrodesis must be performed to correct deformity secondary to a neuromuscular cause. Neuromuscular abnormality will exist as an unrelenting deforming cause. Therefore, fusion must be attempted to prevent recurrence.

When inadequate flexion strength at the MPJ is noted, digital arthrodesis should be considered. Digital arthrodesis acts to strengthen the force of the long flexor tendon. This force is then transmitted to the MPJ, resulting in improved plantar flexion of the joint.[2] In this case, arthrodesis will likely yield more successful long-term results.

Digital fusion also allows for more predictable surgical outcomes. More certain results may be obtained with precise intra-articular positioning and stable fixation. The later influence of additional deforming forces is decreased significantly with fusion of an affected digit. Significant digital deformities addressed with fusion decrease the risk of recurrence.

PROCEDURE

Once the cause has been determined, the surgeon determines if surgical correction is appropriate. The steps in the procedure to correct a hammer toe include resection of the head of the proximal phalanx, extensor digitorum brevis tenotomy, extensor digitorum longus lengthening, first MPJ capsulotomy, and PIPJ arthrodesis. It is imperative that the surgeon analyzes the reduction of the deformity after each step in the procedure by performing the Kelikian push-up test in which pressure is applied to the plantar metatarsal area. If the deformity is reduced using this method, the surgeon may opt for closure at this point in the procedure. However, if the deformity is still evident, a digital arthrodesis is then performed.[12]

GENERAL ANATOMY/JOINT EXPOSURE

Once the patient is under intravenous sedation and local anesthesia has been administered, the surgeon's attention is directed toward the deformed digit. A #15 blade is used to make a linear longitudinal incision from just proximal to the MPJ to slightly distal to the PIPJ. The incision is made through the epidermal and dermal layer of tissue, above the level of the extensor tendon, taking care not to disrupt the tendon.

A lazy "S" incision may be chosen to minimize skin contracture at the incision site. The incision is then deepened through subcutaneous tissue, avoiding any neurovascular structures that may be encountered.[12]

To allow exposure to the head of the proximal phalanx, the extensor digitorum longus tendon may be retracted, incised transversely, or lengthened via a Z-plasty. Next, the collateral ligaments are excised, and excess soft tissue from the distal phalanx is removed. The head of the proximal phalanx is then resected at an appropriate level using a sagittal saw or bone cutter. The rough bone edges are then smoothed with a rongeur or rasp. The surgeon must perform a Kelikian push-up test at this time to determine if extensor digitorum brevis tenotomy is necessary. The tendon can be identified just proximal to the MPJ, and a small stab incision is made just medial or lateral to the tendon with a #15 blade. The blade is then placed transversely, directly plantar to the extensor tendon. Next, the blade is turned to face dorsally and the digit is plantar flexed, causing the blade to incise the tendon. The Kelikian push-up test is performed at this time to determine if extensor digitorum longus lengthening is necessary. If adequate correction has not been established at this time, the extensor tendon lengthening is performed via a Z-plasty technique. The tendon will be reapproximated after arthrodesis is completed if that step is deemed appropriate.[12]

If adequate correction has not been achieved following completion of these steps, a PIPJ arthrodesis is performed. If it has not already been done, the extensor digitorum longus is transected transversely or in a "Z" manner, allowing full exposure of the PIPJ. The distal aspect of the proximal phalanx and proximal aspect of the middle phalanx are cleared of any remaining soft tissue attachments. The cartilage of each articular surface is then resected perpendicular to the long axis of each bone to ensure the toe will be in proper alignment once fixated. Appropriate fixation is then done, followed by suturing of the extensor digitorum longus and closure of subcutaneous tissue and, finally, the skin. The toe is then bandaged in the appropriate sterile manner.[12]

ARTHRODESIS TECHNIQUES

The end-to-end arthrodesis procedure, described in detail earlier, is the most commonly performed digital arthrodesis procedure because it results in less digital shortening and is easy to perform.[12] However, the procedure does have its drawbacks. For instance, there is more potential for the distal fragment to rotate in the frontal plane, which may lead to the development of delayed union or nonunion.

Another option is the peg-in-hole procedure, which uses the distal cortex and central cancellous bone of the proximal phalanx to form a peg. This peg portion is then inserted into a hole created by drilling into the intermedullary shaft of the proximal aspect of the middle phalanx, thus preventing the possibility of the distal fragment rotating in the frontal plane. This procedure is technically more difficult and time intensive than the end-to-end procedure. It may also result in more digital shortening than other methods of arthrodesis. There is always the potential for the peg portion to fracture, which may lead to delayed union or nonunion. The advantages, however, are that no internal fixation is required and high rates of fusion are obtained.[11,31]

Digital "V" arthrodesis and box joint arthrodesis are 2 other surgical options in treating flexion deformities of the digits. In the digital "V" arthrodesis, the surgeon makes a "V" cut distally in the articular surfaces of the proximal and distal phalanges.[30] The bones can then be fixated with a K-wire. Box joint arthrodesis is performed by resecting the inferior aspect of the head of the proximal phalanx and the superior aspect of the base of the middle phalanx. The bones are then fixated appropriately. These procedures are generally performed based on the comfort level and success rates of the surgeon because the clinical complications are similar.[11]

METHODS OF FIXATION
K-Wire

Once the surgeon has determined that arthrodesis is necessary and has completed the steps outlined earlier, fixation can be applied. K-wire fixation remains one of the most popular methods of fixation (**Fig. 3**). This is performed first by aiming a double-ended K-wire through the base of the middle phalanx. The K-wire is then extended distally through the middle and distal phalanges, exiting from the distal aspect of the digit. Careful attention is paid not to disrupt the nail bed. Once the proximal end of the K-wire meets with the articular surface of the PIPJ, it is aimed proximally in a retrograde fashion toward the head of the proximal phalanx, and is then drilled until it meets the subchondral bone in the base of the proximal phalanx. The distal end of the K-wire is then bent and capped to ensure safety.[32]

Although K-wire fixation is technically simple for the surgeon to perform, it has several drawbacks. Pin tract infections are possible as a result of exposure of the distal pin. Psychologically, the patient may be affected by the aesthetics of the hardware. K-wires also do not provide compression between the 2 bone fragments and may allow for proximal migration of the distal fragment; this may lead to delayed union or nonunion of the bones. Bending or breakage of the K-wire is another complication that may be encountered.

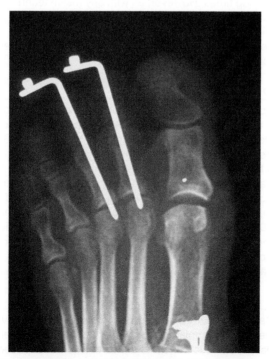

Fig. 3. Radiographic view of DIPJ and PIPJ fusion via K-wire.

Screw and Plate Fixation

Cannulated screws have become an increasingly popular method of digital arthrodesis fixation. Screw fixation allows for compression, which leads to faster healing. Caterini and colleagues[33] found that screw fixation had an arthrodesis rate of 94%. Although the risk of infection always exists, there is no risk for pin tract infection because the hardware remains internal.

There are several fusion techniques using cannulated screws. One technique spares the distal IPJ, with the screw only going across the PIPJ. In this procedure, the distal IPJ is cleared of soft tissue attachments and a guide wire is directed medially from the distal IPJ, through the middle and proximal phalanges. Adequate countersinking must be performed in the distal phalanx to prevent pain occurring at the interphalangeal level. A cannulated screw is then placed into the middle and proximal phalanges, making sure adequate compression is achieved. The guide wire is then removed. Good and Fiala[34] noted development of mallet toe secondary to this form of fixation. This complication is likely because of the absence of any fixation at the distal IPJ. This may lead the surgeon to opt for a different surgical technique.

Another technique using cannulated screws includes the distal IPJ as part of the arthrodesis. This technique is performed by directing a guide wire distally across the middle and distal phalanx, with the wire exiting the distal aspect of the digit. Next, it is directed in a retrograde fashion across the proximal phalanx. A small stab incision is made at the distal aspect of the toe so that the screw can be placed with ease. The screw is then inserted distally to proximally across the distal, middle, and proximal phalanges.[34]

Advantages of screw fixation include maintenance of compression, high fusion rates, and faster healing times. However, as with any fusion technique, complications may occur, such as breakage or movement of the fixation device, painful hardware, floating toe, or a digit that is too straight.[34]

Although the use of plates is off-label, this form of fixation may be an alternative to more traditional screws (**Fig. 4**).

Absorbable Fixation for Digital Arthrodesis

Another option in digital fusion that is becoming more popular amongst surgeons is absorbable fixation devices. Use of absorbable fixation avoids hardware removal at a later date. Available absorbable fixation devices include OrthoSorb pins (DePuy Orthopedics, Warsaw, IN, USA), Nexa Pins (Nexa Orthopedics, San Diego, CA, USA) (**Fig. 5**), and the Inion OTPS Pin System (Inion Inc, Oklahoma City, OK, USA).

OrthoSorb pins are made of poly-p-dioxanone, which is absorbed by the body in 6 months by the process of hydrolysis. Konkel and colleagues[35] found that 73% of their patients had complete fusion with the OrthoSorb pin. This same study showed a success rate of 91%, as determined by the American Orthopaedic Foot and Ankle Society Lesser Toe Scale. The Inion OTPS Pin System is made of polylactic acid and trimethylene carbonate polymers. Absorption of this product begins between 18 and 36 weeks after placement. It subsequently loses strength in 2 to 4 years.

Implant Devices

Several lesser interphalangeal intramedullary implant devices have recently been introduced. In general, these implants boast several advantages over more traditional fixation techniques. An obvious benefit is the elimination of exposed hardware. This proves more convenient and comfortable for the patient while also reducing the risk

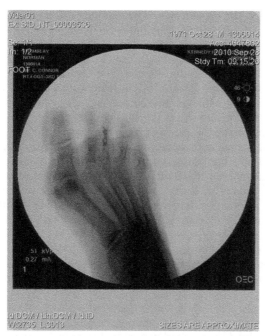

Fig. 4. Third PIPJ maintained via plate fusion, an alternate PIPJ fixation option.

of infection. In addition, implantation avoids the need for violation of healthy joint surfaces. However, these implant devices are significantly more costly than traditional K-wire fixation, one disadvantage that must be kept in mind by the surgeon.[36]

The SMART TOE (Memometal Inc, Memphis, TN, USA) implant was originally designed by Memometal but has recently been acquired by Stryker. This intramedullary memory implant is composed of nitinol, a metal alloy of nickel and titanium, owing to its shape-memory effect. This anchor-shaped implant is available in a standard neutral orientation or a 10° angled design. Following the standard technique of PIPJ exposure and resection, appropriate-sized reamers and broaches are used to prepare

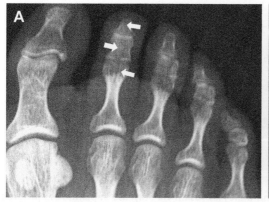
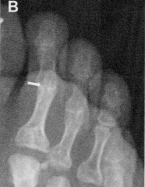

Fig. 5. (A, B) PIPJ fusion via Nexa Pin. Note the arrows outlining the course of the pin.

the medullary canals. The implant should be stored at 0°C for 2 hours before surgery. After preparation of the joint, the implant may be removed from the freezer, allowing for a work time of approximately 1.5 to 2.0 minutes before expansion. Using forceps the proximal portion of the implant is fully seated in the medullary canal of the proximal phalanx. The IPJ is then manually reduced, and the distal legs of the implant are secured within the medullary portion of the middle phalanx. On warming to body temperature, the implant expands, securing it in place. With transverse expansion, the total length of the implant shortens, allowing increased compression across the joint. Benefits specific to this implant include a 1-piece implant design. This eliminates the connection difficulties sometimes encountered in 2-piece implant systems. In addition, SMART TOE's compressive feature may aid in reduced rates of nonunion. The implant's unique anchor shape resists rotation, thus maintaining long-term digital alignment. A recent study by Delmi[37] reviewed 128 patient outcomes after SMART TOE implantation. A total of 170 hammer toe corrections were performed. Of these, 167 toes showed radiologic proximal interphalangeal fusion 12 months postoperatively. Seven total complications were noted, including superficial infection, dislocation of the PIPJ, rupture of implant, and protrusion in the distal IPJ.

The Nexa Orthopedic's StayFuse (Tornier Inc, Stafford, TX, USA) implant is an additional medullary fusion device for correction of hammer toe deformity (**Fig. 6**). This implant is made from a biocompatible titanium material. The implant is in 2 pieces with interlocking male and female counterparts. In addition, the implant is available in a variety of diameters and lengths. Following standard joint exposure and resection, appropriate-sized pilot drills are used to prepare the medullary canals of the opposing

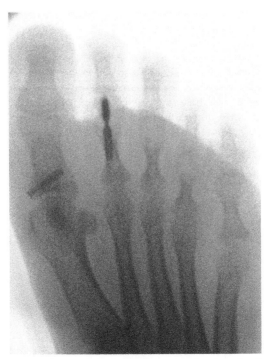

Fig. 6. Radiographic view of second digit PIPJ fusion via StayFuse implant. Also pictured is third digit PIPJ fusion via Nexa Pin fixation.

surfaces of the proximal and middle phalanges. The appropriate-sized StayFuse female component is then driven into the proximal phalanx, followed by insertion of the male component into the middle phalanx. Following reduction of the joint, the hexes of the implant halves are carefully aligned and snapped in place, verifying engagement of the StayFuse implant device. Ellington and colleagues[36] reviewed the outcome of 27 patients undergoing hammer toe correction via StayFuse implantation. A total of 38 toes were fused using this implant. With a mean follow-up of 31 months, union occurred in 23 of 38 (61%) toes. Overall alignment was successfully maintained in 82% of the patients. Complications included nonunion, hardware failure, intraoperative fracture, recurrent deformity with the need for metatarsophalangeal surgery or larger implant.

Wright Medical's Pro-Toe (Wright Medical, Arlington, TN, USA) hammer toe fixation system (**Figs. 7–9**) consists of a 1-piece stainless steel V-shaped blade-screw implant. Four implant options are available. The implant is produced in 2 sizes (small and large) and 2 angle configurations (straight 0° and angled 10°). Following standard joint exposure and resection, the appropriate-sized implant is selected. The medullary canals of the proximal and middle phalanx are then predrilled. To prepare for blade insertion into the middle phalanx, a broach is used to create an opening for the implant. Using the appropriate driver, the implant is driven down the center of the intramedullary canal of the proximal phalanx. The digit is then reduced, and the blade portion of the implant is inserted into the broached canal of the middle phalanx. Neither StayFuse nor Pro-Toe depend on temperature-dependent shape memory, thus eliminating time constraints of implant insertion. Like StayFuse, an

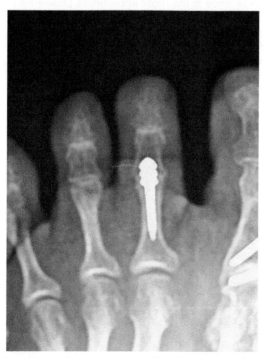

Fig. 7. Pro-Toe implant illustrating proper medullar placement with correction of digital deformity.

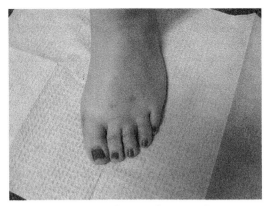

Fig. 8. Postoperative condition 6 weeks after PIPJ fusion with Pro-Toe implant. Incision sites are well healed with maintenance of correction.

additional benefit of Pro-Toe is its 1-piece implant design, thus eliminating the technical difficulty of 2-piece implants.

POSTOPERATIVE COURSE

Postoperative course following digital arthrodesis is ultimately left to the discretion of the surgeon, although the course is highly determined by the choice of fixation technique. Immediately after the operation, the toes should be bandaged in a corrected position. A stiff surgical shoe is the most appropriate choice for postoperative shoe wear. If fixation is provided via K-wire placement across the MPJ, patient ambulation should remain protected. Care should be taken to avoid deformity and stress at the level of the joint. If K-wire fixation does not cross the MPJ, patient activity may be less guarded. Wires should be kept clean and dry to avoid pin tract infection.

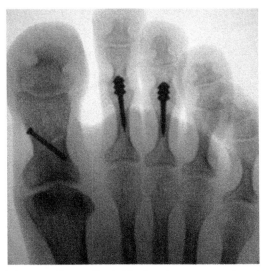

Fig. 9. Associated intraoperative radiograph showing proper placement and alignment within the medullary canal.

Additional forms of fixation may mandate particular postoperative weight-bearing status. However, average postoperative course allows for weight bearing to heel with the use of crutches as needed. Mild analgesics may be provided for pain management. The patient should be instructed to ice and elevate the surgical extremity. Serial radiographs should be obtained to evaluate for osseous consolidation across the PIPJ. K-wires may be removed when radiographic signs of fusion are present, usually approximately 4 to 6 weeks postoperatively.

COMPLICATIONS

As with all lower extremity surgeries, a thorough history and physical examination should be completed to evaluate for potential risk factors and comorbidities that may lead to postoperative complications. Generalized postoperative complications may be attributable to several nonmodifiable risk factors, including diabetes mellitus, rheumatoid arthritis, collagen vascular disease, and osteoporosis, all of which may be responsible for infection, delayed union, nonunion, and impaired wound healing. These risk factors must be recognized and the patient thoroughly educated on the increased risk involved with proceeding with surgery. Modifiable risk factors include tobacco and alcohol abuse, nutritional deficiencies, and patient compliance. These factors must be addressed before proceeding with surgery in an attempt to reduce possible postoperative complications.[38]

Arthrodesis is often seen as an effective surgical approach to correct digital deformity. It is specifically related to a decreased risk of recurrence and more predictable postoperative results.[11] However, general complications are noted, including nonunion, displacement, hardware failures, prolonged swelling, and infections. According to Baig and Geary,[39] distal IPJ instability or deformity is noted with 21% of toes 6 months after surgery. Coughlin[40] observed that 13% of patients developed hyperextension deformity of the PIPJ 5 years after arthrodesis. In addition, he noted that 23% of toes lacked ground contact with the toe pulp.

There are several complications specific to the newer intramedullary implant devices. As with any implant, there is a potential for foreign body–type reactions. Acute or latent infection may also develop secondary to biofilm formation.[38] Excessive postoperative swelling may develop because of increased manipulation, operating time, and surgical trauma. In addition, implantation is more technically demanding than traditional K-wire fixation, leading to incidences of fracture of the proximal or middle phalanges during insertion. If hardware failure occurs, implant devices can be difficult to remove.[41] A specific concern of the authors is the increased rigidity of these devices. As per Wolff's law, bone at the operative site adapts to increased stresses developed secondary to implant placement. However, these rigid implants produce a static lever arm that may not be able to adapt to the surrounding bony architecture. Increased stresses may in turn lead to hardware failure. According to Bayod and colleagues,[42] who performed a finite elements model analysis with PIPJ, fusion, traction, and compression stresses are generally much higher at the proximal and middle phalanges postoperatively.

ALTERNATIVE PROCEDURES

Several adjunctive or alternative procedures may be used to treat significant lesser digit deformities. It is imperative that the surgeon fully understands the causes of variable patient digital deformities. More advanced contractures may involve a degree of deformity at the MPJ. Failure to address additional points of deformity may lead to recurrence of symptoms. Although a flexor to extensor tendon transfer may be indicated for flexible deformities, this procedure may also be appropriate to provide additional stability when used in conjunction with digital arthrodesis procedures. Flexor tendon transfer may replace the loss of intrinsic muscular function, thus augmenting flexion at the MPJ and resisting extension at the IPJ. Transfer of the flexor tendons allows for maintenance of correction along with increased stability of the MPJ. These benefits may in turn assist in plantar plate repair, correction of transverse and sagittal plane deformities, maintenance of toe purchase, and elimination of the positional deforming force in mallet toe deformities.[43] Bayod and colleagues[42] relate a significant correction of deformity using flexor digitorum longus transposition to the dorsal aspect of the proximal phalanx, reducing the maximal dorsal displacement of the proximal phalanx head from 7.28 to 2.89 mm. This study relates similar effectiveness when flexor digitorum brevis is transposed to the dorsal aspect of the proximal phalanx, reducing the maximal dorsal displacement of the proximal phalanx head from 7.28 to 3.52 mm. If there is significant fixed deformity at the level of the MPJ, consideration should be given to alternative procedures, including distal metatarsal osteotomies (Weil osteotomy) and metatarsal head resection. Digital amputation may also be deemed an appropriate surgical alternative for the treatment of severe painful hammer toe deformity. Particularly in the elderly, amputation provides a simple procedure with less morbidity than forefoot reconstruction. In a study of 12 patients (mean age, 78 years), Gallentine and DeOrio[44] assessed the outcome after amputation to address second digit deformity. With an average follow-up of 33 months, 10 patients were satisfied and 2 were satisfied with reservations. A high level of patient satisfaction reveals the value of digital amputation as an alternative to more complex reconstructive procedures.

HALLUX INTERPHALANGEAL ARTHRODESIS
Historical Background

Fusion of the hallux IPJ has been used for more than a century to provide relief from pain in patients with deformities at that level.[45] Podiatrists and orthopedists commonly perform this procedure in conjunction with metatarsophalangeal procedures or as an unaccompanied procedure for the treatment of a multitude of ailments.

Numerous types of fixation have been used to obtain union of the head of the proximal phalanx and the base of the distal phalanx of the hallux. As far back as 1980, Shives and Johnson[46] advocated the use of intramedullary screws to achieve fusion of the hallux IPJ. This technique is still popular today; however, patient selection is important when using this method of fixation.

Many investigators such as Mann[47] and Jahss[48] have had a great deal of success using K-wires, despite the ease with which surgeons now use screw fixation to gain arthrodesis. K-wires are an excellent choice in patients who are not good candidates for screw fixation, such as those with poor bone stock. Osteopenia may be seen in a wide variety of patients, in particular the elderly population and those with systemic arthritides.

Sharon and McClain[49] published an article in 1985 that listed a miniature fixator as an option for fusing the IPJ of the hallux. Although not commonly performed because of the general complications that are encountered with any external fixator, such as surgeon error and high infection rates, this method has been used historically to achieve fusion at the level of the hallux IPJ.

Indications

Arthrodesis of the hallux IPJ is used to treat a variety of maladies that lead to pain and instability. The most common indication for arthrodesis of the hallux IPJ is deformity.

Numerous deformities exist at the level of the hallux IPJ in large part, because of structural abnormalities of the foot itself, such as cavus foot.[50] A foot that is plantar flexed puts a large amount of pressure on the forefoot, leading the toes, including the hallux, to act as stabilizers against the ground. As a result, the flexor tendons overpower the extensor tendons, leading to flexion deformities at the IPJ.[50,51] Other causes of deformity at this joint level are hallux abducto valgus, iatrogenic or congenital hallux varus, sesamoidectomy, and degenerative or posttraumatic arthritis. Less common causes of muscle imbalances of the hallux IPJ include Charcot-Marie-Tooth disease and postpolio syndrome. Arthrodesis of the hallux IPJ can also be used as an adjunctive procedure to a Jones tenosuspension.[50]

Few contraindications exist for hallux IPJ arthrodesis. Infection in the bone, severe osteoporosis, or advanced peripheral vascular disease should lead the surgeon to use more conservative options.

Physical Examination

As with any patient, determining whether fusion of the hallux IPJ is an appropriate surgical option should only be decided after a thorough history and physical examination. Most importantly, the physician must establish whether the patient has adequate blood supply to heal an incision located in the most distal aspect of the forefoot. The surgeon may check for dorsalis pedis and posterior tibial pulses, capillary fill time, and pedal hair as indicators for sufficient circulation to the extremities. If there is any question regarding the circulatory status of the patient, ankle-brachial indices may be obtained before proceeding.

Next, the hallux IPJ should be put through range-of-motion tests to determine the degree of the deformity. The range of motion of the first MPJ must also be assessed. According to Alexander,[51] if the MPJ cannot be plantar flexed to at least the neutral position, surgery at that level should be performed in conjunction with fusion of the hallux IPJ.

Radiographs should be obtained before surgical planning. Weight-bearing dorsoplantar, lateral, and medial oblique images must all be examined to determine the best operative course for the patient. The surgeon should examine the length of the proximal and distal phalanges, the hallux abductus angle, the amount of arthroses at the level of the joint, and signs of osteopenia such as poor cortical definition.[52] The patient's bone stock helps to determine the type of fixation that will lead to fusion of the joint.

Surgical Technique

Many different incisions may be performed to gain exposure to the IPJ. The incision options can be transverse semielliptical, longitudinal linear, curvilinear, or T shaped. Another incision that has become popular for this procedure is the serpentine incision, which begins dorsomedially along the proximal phalanx, is carried over the center aspect of the IPJ, and continues distal laterally. Incision planning should be determined based on the procedure and fixation that are being performed.[50,52] Incisions are typically made on the dorsum of the hallux, although a plantar incision is a viable option.

On completion of the skin incision, the incision should next be carried to the subcutaneous level until the extensor tendons can be identified. The extensor hallucis longus should be incised transversely and reflected proximally and distally so visualization of the hallux IPJ is established. The amount of bone that is removed from the head of the proximal phalanx and the base of the distal phalanx should be determined based on the quality of the articular cartilage and the amount of correction that is needed at the joint. It is at the discretion of the surgeon whether a power saw or bone cutter is necessary for resection of the articular cartilage. The bone is cut so that the hallux IPJ is in a neutral position, with no deviation in the sagittal or transverse plane. Derner and Meyr[45] have suggested making a V-shaped osteotomy in both bones, with the convex "V" being the base of the distal phalanx and the concave "V" being the head of the proximal phalanx. A high level of frontal plane stability may be achieved with this form of fixation. The maximum amount of contact should be made between the 2 bones to ensure fusion. Smooth bone edges are more likely to undergo nonunion or malunion. Some investigators advocate subchondral drilling of the distal phalanx to stimulate revascularization.[52]

Fixation

There are many options available for fixation of the hallux IPJ. K-wires, monofilament wire, staples, plates, and screws are all fixation options available for establishing arthrodesis of the hallux. This article provides a brief overview of the fixation methods available.

K-wires

Two crossing K-wires provide stabilization of the hallux IPJ. Depending on patient factors such as height, weight, and bone stock, 1.1 mm (0.045 in) or 1.6 mm (0.062 in) K-wires can be used. On removing the articular cartilage of the distal and proximal phalanges, an antegrade drill hole is made in the central portion of the base of the distal phalanx in a superior position. The second K-wire is placed at the base of the distal phalanx in a slightly inferior position to avoid striking the first K-wire. The wires are then retrograded to the distal tip of the distal phalanx. Before driving the wires into the proximal phalanx, the distal phalanx must be placed in a neutral position with regard to sagittal and transverse plane motion. The wires are then driven in a proximal direction through the medial and lateral cortices of the proximal phalanx, respectively. Static stabilization of the fusion site occurs when driving the K-wires into the proximal phalanx. The K-wires should then be bent parallel to one another using a wire bender or Frazier suction. Any excess wire should then be cut and the ends capped. Before closure of the incision, MPJ range of motion should be assessed to ensure that the K-wires have not penetrated this joint. The extensor tendons should then be reapproximated using a suture material of the surgeons choosing. The skin is then closed with sutures.[50,52]

Screw fixation

Several different screws have been used for fixation of the hallux IPJ. One cancellous lag screw (**Fig. 10**) or one fully threaded cortical screw can be used to achieve fusion. When the surgeon is in doubt about the stabilization of one screw for fixation, a K-wire can be used to increase rotational stability. However, one screw may be adequate. The most commonly used size of cancellous lag screws for hallux IPJ arthrodesis is 4 mm.[50] Before insertion of the screw, a 2-mm drill bit is used to predrill the distal phalanx. A small stab incision is made at the distal tip of the hallux, and the 4-mm cancellous lag screw is driven across the distal and proximal phalanges. One can also use a cannulated 4-mm screw, and, in this instance, a pin is used for temporary fixation before advancing the permanent screw. The guide wire is then removed. If the fixation of choice is a 3.5-mm cortical screw, a 3.5-mm glide hole is made in the distal phalanx. This creates the overdrill that will lead to compression when the 3.5-mm screw is inserted. The screw is then inserted.[50,51]

Alternative Options of Fixation

Although the most commonly used methods of fixation are screws and K-wires, some other techniques are worth mentioning. Staples may be a good option for stabilizing

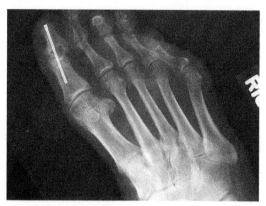

Fig. 10. Intra-articular comminuted fracture through the base of the distal phalanx. Screw fixation used to perform primary interphalangeal arthrodesis.

the proximal and distal phalanges because they are bendable and can be manipulated to gain adequate bony contact and therefore fusion. Monofilament wire is an early technique that is now less commonly used, although still a valid means of hallux IPJ fusion. A variety of plates and screws can also be used; however, because of the limited surface area of the distal and proximal phalanges of the hallux, this may not be feasible in all patients and a backup method of fixation should be planned.

Postoperative Management

On completion of the surgical procedure, a dry sterile dressing is applied to the incision site. The first postoperative dressing change can be performed at 1 week. Swelling needs to be kept to a minimum, and the patient should be advised to ice and elevate the foot. A surgical shoe will be dispensed to the patient, and, depending on the method of fixation used, the patient will likely remain non–weight bearing for at least 6 weeks. Some surgeons believe that immediate weight bearing to tolerance is acceptable; however, if this is desired, the hallux should be splinted for 6 weeks. Patients with K-wire fixation may need to be non–weight bearing for a longer period than a patient with screw fixation because K-wires only provide static stabilization and can be easily disrupted. Radiographs should be taken at 3, 6, and 9 weeks to monitor for signs of fusion. Once bony union is established, fixation may be removed. Screws can be a permanent means of fixation; however, if hardware irritation occurs, they can be removed. K-wires may be removed in an office setting once hallux interphalangeal arthrodesis has been achieved.[52]

Complications

Nonunion is a complication that leads to recurrence or worsening of the deformity of the hallux. Adequate blood supply, insufficient bony apposition, improper fixation, and early ambulation lead to nonunion and should be avoided when possible. There is a possibility of rotation if one screw is used as fixation, which may lead to malposition of the hallux. Some other complications that may be encountered are migration of screws or K-wires, dehiscence of the incision site, infection, osteomyelitis, and necrosis.

DISCUSSION

Arthrodesis has long been performed on both the hallux and lesser digits. A multitude of digital deformities may be successfully addressed via IPJ fusion. The present-day surgeon has many options regarding arthrodesis technique and fixation. Once the cause of deformity is determined, an educated decision may be made regarding the proper surgical approach. Patient factors and surgeon preference likely determine which method of fixation is utilized for correction. Digital arthrodesis has proved to be a reliable method of digital correction. However, as with all surgical procedures, the potential exists for complications. Careful preoperative planning, precise surgical technique, and strict postoperative care may greatly reduce the risk of complications.

ACKNOWLEDGMENTS

The authors would like to thank Elyann Doebler, DPM, and Joseph Mirarchi, DPM.

REFERENCES

1. Soule RE. Operation for the correction of hammer toe. N Y Med J 1910;84: 649–50.
2. Schuberth J. Hammer toe syndrome. J Foot Ankle Surg 1999;38(2):166–78.
3. Young CS. An operation for the correction of hammer toe and claw toe. J Bone Joint Surg 1938;20:715–9.
4. Taylor RG. An operative procedure for the treatment of hammer toe and claw toe. J Bone Joint Surg 1940;22:608–9.
5. Selig S. Hammer toe: a new procedure for its correction. Surg Gynecol Obstet 1941;72:101–5.
6. Thomas J. Diagnosis and treatment of forefoot disorders. Section 1: digital deformities clinical practice guideline forefoot disorders panel. J Foot Ankle Surg 2009; 42(2).
7. Coughlin MJ, Pinsonneault T. Operative treatment of interdigital neuroma. A long-term follow-up study. J Bone Joint Surg Am 2001;83(9):1321–8.
8. Coughlin MJ, Schenck RC Jr, Shurnas PS, et al. Concurrent interdigital neuroma and MTP joint instability: long-term results of treatment. Foot Ankle Int 2002; 23(11):1017–25.
9. Lehman DE, Smith RW. Radiographic analysis of proximal interphalangeal joint arthrodesis with an intramedullary fusion device for lesser toe deformities. Foot Ankle Int 1995;16(9):535–41.
10. Coughlin MJ, Dorris J, Polk E. Operative repair of the fixed hammer toe deformity. Foot Ankle Int 2000;21(2):94–104.
11. Lehman DE, Smith RW. Treatment of symptomatic hammer toe with a proximal interphalangeal joint arthrodesis. Foot Ankle Int 1995;16(9):535–41.
12. McGlamry ED. Lesser ray deformities. In: MacAulay R, editor. Comprehensive textbook of foot surgery. Baltimore (MD): Williams & Wilkins; 1978. p. 253–372.
13. Mann RA, Coughlin MJ. Lesser toe deformities. Instr Course Lect 1987;36: 137–59.
14. Schrier J, Verheyen C, Louwerens J. Definitions of hammer toe and claw toe. An evaluation of the literature. J Am Podiatr Med Assoc 2009;99(3):194–7.
15. Coughlin MJ. Subluxation and dislocation of the second metatarsophalangeal joint. Orthop Clin N Am 1989;20(4):535–51.
16. Coughlin MJ. Second metatarsophalangeal joint instability in the athlete. Foot Ankle 1993;14(6):309–19.
17. Brahms MA. Common foot problems. J Bone Joint Surg Am 1967;49(8):1653–64.

18. Brahms MA. The small toes. In: Jahss M, editor. Disorders of the foot and ankle. Philadelphia: WB Saunders; 1991. p. 1187.
19. Coughlin MJ. Operative repair of the mallet toe deformity. Foot Ankle Int 1995; 16(3):109–16.
20. Mizel MS. Anatomy and pathophysiology of the lesser toes. In: Gould J, editor. Operative foot surgery. Philadelphia: WB Saunders; 1993. p. 84–5.
21. Richardson E. Lesser toe abnormalities. In: Crenshaw AH, editor. Campbell's operative orthopaedics. 8th edition. St Louis (MO): Mosby; 1992. p. 2742–4.
22. Ross ER, Menelaus MB. Open flexor tenotomy for hammer toes and curly toes in childhood. J Bone Joint Surg Br 1984;66(5):770–1.
23. Sweetnam R. Congenital curly toes: an investigation into the value of treatment. Lancet 1958;2(7043):397–400.
24. Myerson MS, Shereff MJ. The pathological anatomy of claw and hammer toes. J Bone Joint Surg Am 1989;71(1):45–9.
25. Hamer AJ, Stanley D, Smith TW. Surgery for curly toe deformity: a double-blind, randomised, prospective trial. J Bone Joint Surg Br 1993;75(4):662–3.
26. Boc SF, Martone JD. Varus toes: a review and case report. J Foot Ankle Surg 1995;34(2):220–2.
27. Angirasa AK, Augoyard M, Coughlin MJ, et al. Hammer toe, mallet toe, and claw toe. Foot Ankle Spec 2011;4(3):182–7.
28. Lapidus PW. Operation for correction of hammer toe. J Bone Joint Surg 1939;21: 977–82.
29. Mann RA, Coughlin MJ. Lesser toe deformities. In: Jahss M, editor. Disorders of the foot and ankle. Philadelphia: WB Saunders; 1991. p. 1207–9.
30. Pichney GA, Derner R, Lauf E. Digital "V" arthrodesis. J Foot Ankle Surg 1993; 32(5):473–9.
31. Lamm BM, Ribeiro CE, Vlahovic TC, et al. Lesser proximal interphalangeal joint arthrodesis: a retrospective analysis of the peg in hole and end to end procedures. J Am Podiatr Med Assoc 2001;91(7):331–6.
32. Edwards WH, Beischer AD. Interphalangeal joint arthrodesis of the lesser toes. Foot Ankle Clin 2003;7:43–8.
33. Caterini R, Farsetti P, Tarantino U, et al. Arthrodesis of the toe joints with an intramedullary cannulated screw for correction of hammertoe deformity. Foot Ankle Int 2004;25(4):256–61.
34. Good J, Fiala K. Digital surgery: current trends and techniques. Clin Podiatr Med Surg 2010;27:583–99.
35. Konkel KF, Menger AG, Retzlaff SA. Hammertoe correction using an absorbable intramedullary pin. Foot Ankle Int 2007;28(8):916–20.
36. Ellington JK, Anderson RB, Davis WH. Radiographic analysis of proximal interphalangeal joint arthrodesis with an intramedullary fusion device for lesser toe deformities. Foot Ankle Int 2010;31(5):372–6.
37. Delmi M. Hammer toe surgical correction. Available at: http://www.mmi-usa.com/pdf/hammertoe.pdf. Accessed July 5, 2011.
38. Bibbo C, Jaffe L, Goldkind A. Complications of digital and lesser metatarsal surgery. Clin Podiatr Med Surg 2010;27:485–507.
39. Baig AU, Geary NP. Fusion rate and patient satisfaction in proximal interphalangeal joint fusion of the minor toes using Kirschner wire fixation. The Foot 1996;6:120–1. Available at: http://dx.doi.org/10.1016/S0958-2592(96)90003-6. Accessed July 5, 2011.
40. Coughlin MJ. Lesser toe abnormalities. J Bone Joint Surg Am 2002;84:1446–69.

41. Yu GV, Vincent AL, Khoury WE, et al. Techniques of digital arthrodesis: revisiting the old and discovering the new. Clin Podiatr Med Surg 2004;21:17–50.

42. Bayod J, Losa-Iglesias M, Becerro de Bengoa-Vallejo R, et al. Advantages and drawbacks of proximal interphalangeal joint fusion versus flexor tendon transfer in the correction of hammer and claw toe deformity. A finite-element study. J Biomech Eng 2010;132:051002-1–051002-7.

43. Slavitt J. Balancing digital arthrodesis with flexor tendon transfers and MPJ corrections. Podiatry Today 2011;24(3):36–40.

44. Gallentine JW, DeOrio JK. Removal of the second toe for severe hammertoe deformity in elderly patients. Foot Ankle Int 2005;26(5):353–8.

45. Dermer RI, Meyr AN. Hallux interphalangeal joint arthrodesis. J Foot Ankle Surg 2009;48(3):408–10.

46. Shives TC, Johnson KA. Arthrodesis of the hallux interphalangeal joint of the great toe—an improved technique. Foot Ankle 1980;1(1):26–9.

47. Mann RA. Arthrodesis of the foot and ankle. In: Mann RA, Coughlin MJ, editors. Surgery of the foot and ankle, vol. 1. 6th edition. St Louis (MO): Mosby-Year Book; 1993. p. 712.

48. Jahss MH. Disorders of the first ray. In: Jahss MH, editor. Disorders of the foot and ankle. 2nd edition. Philadelphia: WB Saunders; 1991. p. 1139.

49. Sharon MC, McClain J. An alternative fixation technique when performing hallux interphalangeal joint fusions. J Foot Surg 1985;24:132.

50. McGlamry ED. Comprehensive textbook of foot surgery. Baltimore (MD): Williams & Wilkins; 1987. p. 648–50.

51. Alexander IJ. Hallux interphalangeal arthrodesis. In: Kitaoka HB, editor. Master techniques in orthopedic surgery: the foot and ankle. 2nd edition. Philadelphia: Lippincott Williams & Wilkins; 2002. p. 19–26.

52. Yu GV, Vargo FE, Brook JW. Arthrodesis of the interphalangeal joint of the hallux: a simple and effective technique. J Am Podiatr Med Assoc 2001;91(8):427–34.

First Metatarsophalangeal Joint Arthrodesis

Robert M. Rajczy, DPM[a], Patrick R. McDonald, DPM[a,b],
Howard S. Shapiro, DPM[c,*], Steven F. Boc, DPM[d,e]

KEYWORDS

• First metatarsophalangeal joint • Arthrodesis • Hallux
• Salvage arthrodesis

Arthrodesis of the first metatarsophalangeal joint (MTPJ) is used primarily for end-stage hallux rigidus whereby pain, crepitus, and limitation of motion is noted at the joint. Arthrodesis at the first MTPJ also has it uses as a primary procedure for rheumatoid arthritis when severe deformity is present, as well as for salvage procedures for failed joint arthroplasties with or without implant, fractures with intra-articular extension, avascular necrosis, and infection management. Despite variances in candidacy and technique, the ultimate goal is the same. A purpose-driven first MTPJ arthrodesis should provide stable fixation, attain suitable positioning for a reasonable gait, maintain adequate length, and create a stable platform for a plantigrade foot type. The purpose of course is the elimination of pain with ambulation.

ANATOMY

The first MTPJ is composed of the articular surface from the base of the proximal phalanx of the hallux, which is concave, and the articular surface of the head of the first metatarsal, which is convex. The head of the first metatarsal differs from those of the lesser metatarsals in that it has two grooves separated by a central crest plantarly to accommodate two sesamoid bones. The joint is considered an ellipsoid joint.[1]

The joint is surrounded by a fibrous capsule, which extends more proximal plantarly than dorsally. Ligaments associated with the joint are the plantar metatarsophalangeal ligament, the medial and lateral metatarsal sesamoid ligaments, the intersesamoid ligament, and collateral ligaments.[1]

[a] Hahnemann University Hospital, Philadelphia, PA, USA
[b] Private Practice, Mountain Valley Orthopedic, P.C, East Stroudsburg, PA, USA
[c] Hahnemann University Hospital, Podiatric Medicine and Surgery Programme, Philadelphia, PA, USA
[d] Podiatric Medicine and Surgery Residency Program, Hahnemann University Hospital, 235 North, Broad Street, Suite 300, Philadelphia, PA 19107, USA
[e] Department of Surgery, Drexel University, College of Medicine, Philadelphia, PA, USA
* Corresponding author. Hahnemann University Hospital, 235 North Broad Street, Suite 300, Philadelphia, PA 19107.
E-mail address: poddytrained@gmail.com

Clin Podiatr Med Surg 29 (2012) 41–49
doi:10.1016/j.cpm.2011.11.001
0891-8422/12/$ – see front matter © 2012 Elsevier Inc. All rights reserved.

Blood supply is from the first dorsal and plantar arteries or their medial digital branches, depending at which level the arteries divide. Innervation is from the medial terminal branch of the deep peroneal nerve, medial dorsal cutaneous nerve, and medial plantar nerve.[1]

BIOMECHANICS

The first MTPJ is capable of flexion-extension and adduction-abduction as well as longitudinal rotation.

During ambulation the joint is in a neutral position or slightly dorsiflexed during most of the stance phase. In late stance the joint reaches a peak of 50° to 60° of extension and remains at 30° to 40° of extension throughout the swing phase. The sesamoids move anteriorly with joint extension and posteriorly with joint plantarflexion.

HALLUX LIMITUS AND RIGIDUS
Etiology

Hallux limitus is the term used to define a progressive pathology of the first MTPJ with limited dorsiflexion in the sagittal plane. Traditionally the restricted motion in this joint is considered dorsiflexion of less than 65°. Hallux rigidus is a progression of the deformity in which motion in the joint is limited to less than 10° of dorsiflexion.[2] The progression of this condition has prompted various debates as well as classifications in the literature, based predominantly on the combination of clinical and radiographic findings (**Table 1**). Causes of this deformity include increased age, female gender, trauma, previous surgery, osteochondritis desiccans, and rheumatoid and other arthropathies.

Several biomechanical factors have been attributed to the progression of this deformity. Root and colleagues described 5 biomechanical causes of hallux limitus including elongated first metatarsal, hypermobility of the first ray, immobilization, degenerative joint disease, and metatarsus primus elevatus.[3] Other biomechanical etiologies including pes planus, metatarsus adductus, long proximal phalanx of the hallux, sesamoid abnormality, tarsal coalition, and hallux valgus (**Box 1**).

Indication for Surgery

First MTPJ arthrodesis has been a mainstay in the treatment of a wide variety first MTPJ disorders. The procedure frequently has been the choice for a definitive solution for degenerative changes of the first MTPJ. Removing damaged articular surfaces and

Table 1
Summary of Regnauld classification[4]

	Clinical Evaluation	Radiographic Evaluation
Grade I	Range of motion (ROM) <40°, dorsiflexion <20° Acute pain	Slight joint space narrowing Flattening of first metatarsal head Mild spurring around joint
Grade II	Arthrosis Limited ROM Intermittent pain Metatarsalgia	Narrowing of joint space Extensive spurring Flattening of metatarsal head Hypertrophy of joint
Grade III	Ankylosis Absent/little ROM Pain with any movement	Loss of joint space Joint mice Hypertrophy of metatarsal, phalanx, sesamoids Periarticular osteophytes

---

Box 1
Etiological factors of hallux limitus/rigidus[5]

1. Biomechanical
   a. Hypermobility
   b. Elongated first ray
   c. Pes planus foot type
   d. Metatarsus adductus
   e. Elongated hallux proximal phalanx
   f. Hallux valgus
   g. Tarsal coalition
2. Arthropathies
   a. Rheumatoid
   b. Gout
3. Trauma
4. Age
5. Congenital
   a. Female gender

---

eliminating motion is a cornerstone of the treatment of chronic osteoarthritis pain in the foot. Chronic joint pain from hallux limitus/rigidus, especially degenerative joint disease categorized in the latter stages, has been treated with surgical fusion. However, it has been debated in the literature whether a total-implant arthroplasty or arthrodesis has a more favorable long-term outcome. Gibson and colleagues evaluated patients 2 years after arthroplasty and arthrodesis surgery, concluding that arthrodesis has fewer postsurgical complications and a higher satisfaction rate among patients.[6] First MTPJ arthrodesis is by no means restricted to symptoms from osteoarthritis. Jenter and colleagues used fusion to treat cerebral palsy–induced hallux valgus with favorable outcomes.[7] Gout, rheumatoid arthritis, and Charcot are also pathologies in which arthrodesis has generated promising results. Finally, arthrodesis has been used for first-ray salvage procedure including failed hallux valgus or MTPJ implant surgery, osteomyelitis, or trauma.[8]

Preoperative Evaluation

Activity level, age, gender, footwear, and profession should be considered when determining the appropriate procedure for correction. Taking a thorough history and physical examination can help in deciding the appropriate procedure. The patient's complaint can also help determine proper procedure. Does the patient have pain with activity when wearing or not wearing shoes, or only from pressure with certain types of footwear? The answers to these questions can help guide the clinician in choosing the appropriate procedure, whether a cheilectomy, joint-sparing procedure, destructive procedures consisting of joint implantation or arthrodesis.[9]

Radiographic assessment should consider joint space, periarticular exostosis, loose bodies, metatarsal position (elevated or rectus), sesamoid apparatus, hallux abductus angle, and rearfoot to forefoot relationship (to assess any functional abnormalities that could play a key role in causing structural abnormalities at the first MTPJ).[9]

Circulation, bone quality, and tobacco use are other factors that play a significant role in the decision to perform an arthrodesis. Patients with diminished circulation or bone quality can have problems such as lengthy fusion times and fixation failures, respectively. These patients may need to be immobilized for longer periods of time, which can lead to other problems such as disuse osteopenia, deep vein thrombosis, and reflex sympathetic dystrophy.[9]

Surgical Technique

Local anesthesia with intravenous sedation is most commonly administered; however, general anesthesia can be used especially for those procedures that can be of greater length, such as revisional fusions. Hemostasis can be accomplished with the use of an ankle or thigh tourniquet. The patient is positioned in the supine position and prepped sterilely. An incision approximately 6 to 7 cm in length is made on the dorsal-medial aspect of the first MTPJ. The incision is carried down to subcutaneous tissue, where all small bleeders are cauterized and all neurovascular structures are retracted from the surgical field. Next, the capsular layer is exposed and transected sharply to expose the first MTPJ. The joint is visualized as well as any exostosis, spurring, and cartilage wear or destruction.

The first metatarsal and proximal phalanx are fixed end to end after periarticular osteophyte resection and cartilaginous destruction. Opposing ends are contoured either manually or with a conical reamer that assures convex-concave articulation with minimal length being sacrificed. Conical reamers also allow for ideal positioning of the hallux without losing bony apposition. The concave remain corresponds with the first metatarsal head. A 0.062 Kirschner wire (K-wire) is placed centrally in the head and parallel with the diaphysis. After the correct size is determined, which should be slightly smaller than the head itself, the reamer is placed over the K-wire and run until subchondral cancellous bone is exposed. The surrounding bone may be excised with a rongeur. Next the base of the proximal phalanx is addressed by using the convex reamer of corresponding size to devoid the concave articulation of all cartilage and expose subchondral cancellous bone. Again, any additional spurring or osteophytes may be removed with a rongeur. 0.062 K-wires are used to drill both sides of the fusion site subchondrally to increase blood flow to the fusion site.

Proper positioning of the great toe should be between 5° and 15° of dorsiflexion with respect to the weight-bearing surface, with 10° to 20° of abduction. There should be no inversion or eversion of the toe. Usually the authors load the foot against a flat surface, such as the top of the hardware being used. The fusion site is then placed into the correct position and temporarily fixed with K-wires until permanent fixation is achieved.

Several fixation methods have been deemed acceptable both in the literature and in practice, not all of which require conical reaming. These techniques include, but are not limited, to a single 3.5 cortical interfragmentary lag screw, crossed 0.062 K-wires, dorsal plating with or without a 3.5 interfragmentary lag screw, or crossing 3.5 interfragmentary lag screws. The crossing screws may be applied starting distally from the medial and lateral sides and crossing, or starting both from the medial side and crossing the fixation site, one distally and one proximally (**Figs. 1** and **2**).

External fixation is a newer approach to fixation of the first MTPJ. The authors commonly use this technique for revisional fusions as well as infection management. Antibiotic beads are placed into the resected area and external fixation is used to maintain the length of the first ray (**Fig. 3**). After infection has cleared, an interpositional bone graft is placed into the deficit. Bone graft can be either autologous or

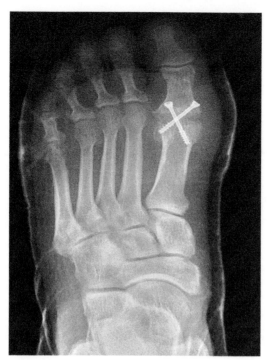

Fig. 1. Immediately postoperative radiograph of crossing 3.5 screw fixation.

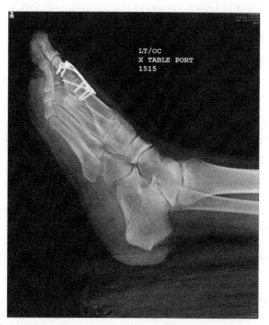

Fig. 2. Immediately postoperative radiograph of arthrodesis with plate and lag screw fixation.

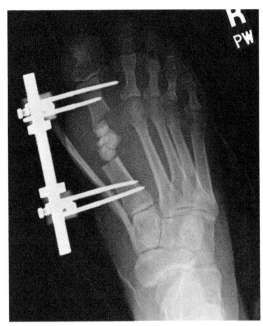

Fig. 3. Postoperative radiograph of MTPJ resection with application of antibiotic beads and external fixator.

allogenic, depending on factors such as deficit size, bone quality, and bone availability.

The wound is closed in layers, repairing the capsule with 2-0 Vicryl and subcutaneous tissue with 3-0 Vicryl, then the skin is sutured with either subcuticular 4-0 Monocryl, reinforced with sterile strips, or 4-0 Prolene.

Postoperative Care

The patient is placed into a below-knee fiberglass cast with distal extension and foot plate past the toes, and is non–weight-bearing for the first 6 weeks. Subsequent cast changes are done after week 1 to assess the incision site for healing and infection. Radiographs are also taken at this time to confirm proper alignment of the joint and that no changes have occurred since the time of procedure. At week 3 the cast is removed along with the sutures. At week 6 further radiographs are taken to ascertain any signs of bony fusion. If there are signs of fusion such as bridging of bone, the patient may be progressed to a cam walker; otherwise he or she is placed back into a hard cast for an additional 2 weeks.

Once bony fusion is noted (usually 8–12 weeks postoperatively), the patient returns to supportive footwear as tolerated, and is started on gentle range of motion of the foot and ankle, avoiding any intentional motion at the first MTPJ (**Fig. 4**). Physical therapy may be undertaken if prolonged immobilization is encountered.

Complications

The most common complications of arthrodesis of the first MTPJ are nonunion and malunion. Nonunion can be caused by several factors such as inadequate fixation, insufficient cartilage resection, and noncompliance by the patient. Malunion can be associated with deviation in one or all planes (transverse, sagittal, and frontal) as

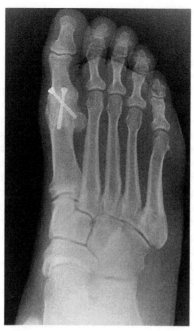

Fig. 4. Eight months after surgery. Bony consolidation is noted through the fusion site, with the crossing screws intact.

well as shortening of the toe, and can pose problems with ambulation that are as bad as or worse than the presenting problem.

SALVAGE BONE-BLOCK ARTHRODESIS
Pathology and Indications

A fusion of the first MTPJ is frequently used as a procedure of last resort. Whether it is an attempt to fuse a joint in end-stage hallux limitus, recover failed first-ray surgery, or treat chronic arthritides, a first MTPJ fusion is a final action aimed at maintaining a functional ambulatory foot. Several different procedures can be used for an arthrodesis, including screw or plate fixation, bone grafts, and external fixation devices. When dealing with certain pathologies, the first MTPJ cannot be fused using conventional fixation. Osteomyelitis, septic arthritis, avascular necrosis, chronic gout, and rheumatoid arthritis may cause bone breakdown of the distal first metatarsal or proximal phalanx. In these circumstances, when bone is no longer viable or infected, resection is warranted to remove all defunct tissue. In certain cases when resection of bone is necessary, the first ray must maintain its anatomic length to maintain a functional ambulatory foot. Bone graft, whether autogenous or allograft, is used most commonly with plating to maintain the length of the first ray. Stapleton and colleagues discussed using an iliac crest graft with a 9-hole plate with an external fixation device to maintain arthrodesis in a patient with chronic gout and osteomyelitis.[10] Brodsky and colleagues used an iliac crest graft with plate fixation following complications of first-ray surgery; results were favorable, with no further breakdown of the joint and with overall satisfaction of hallux alignment and function.[11]

Surgical Principles of Salvage Arthrodesis

The standard for first metatarsal head osteomyelitis has long been aggressive resection with or without hallux amputation. This section discusses a staged approach to first-ray salvage in cases of osteomyelitis. Preceding the final stage of fusion the appropriate areas of infected bone are resected to what is believed clinically to be healthy bone. Resected bone is then sent to both Pathology and Microbiology, as well as clean margins of assumed healthy bone, to confirm negative biological intrusion at this site. From a clinical perspective, it is often one's instinct and has been accepted practice to overresect an area of bone thought to be infected. The purpose of this is clearly to make sure that enough infected bone has been taken so as not be held liable or to have to perform any repeat procedure because of proximal extension of such infection. This methodology might be considered best practice but often seems presumptuous and quite possibly out of line with regard to a patient's best interest. In the authors' experience of resecting only as much bone as what appears to be infected intraoperatively and then taking a clean margin of what is left of hard, white, clinically uninfected bone, the authors have almost never had the specimen return from Pathology with osseous foreign biological growth, and this may be a topic for further research and debate. Regardless, the authors' technique has included this minimalist approach to bone resection along with application of antibiotic beads to prepare the area for a graft-salvage arthrodesis. Shortening of the first ray is a complication of such a procedure, but application of a uniplanar external fixation device can maintain length during postoperative healing and antibiotic management. Following appropriate skin closure, the patient will undergo antibiotic therapy for an appropriate period of time; duration and antibiotic of choice are determined by the results of microbiology and pathology. The patient is placed in a posterior splint with non–weight-bearing status for the postoperative duration.

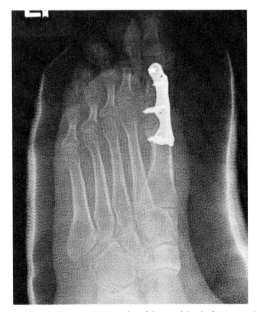

Fig. 5. Immediately postoperative radiograph of bone-block fusion with dorsal screw and plate fixation.

Surgical Approach and Technique

A dorsal medial incision approximately 6 to 8 cm in length is used, possibly following prior incision sites and extending from the distal third of the first metatarsal to the proximal two-thirds of the proximal phalanx. The incision is deepened through the subcutaneous tissues and all neurovascular structures, and the long extensor tendons retracted. At this point, the pins of the external fixator are removed. A linear capsulotomy is performed over the dorsal aspect of the joint, exposing the remaining proximal phalanx and first metatarsal. All nonviable bone is resected from each bone and sent once again to Pathology and Microbiology to rule out osteomyelitis. The area can be once again be pulse lavaged at the surgeon's discretion. At this point, either autogenous or allogeneic graft is shaped to the appropriate size (no >2 cm in length) and inserted into the gap between the first metatarsal and proximal phalanx. Once good alignment and position of the hallux is confirmed, a dorsal plate with locking-screw fixation is used to secure the graft (**Fig. 5**). All hardware placement is confirmed with fluoroscopy. Copious flushing of the incision site is followed by reapproximating the capsule, subcutaneous tissue, and skin. A dry sterile dressing followed by a below-knee non–weight-bearing cast is applied.

REFERENCES

1. Hirsch BE, Minugh-Purvis N. Anatomy of the lower extremity. Arthrology 2002;64–7.
2. Botek G, Anderson MA. Etiology, pathophysiology, and staging of hallux rigidus. Clin Podiatr Med Surg 2011;28(2):229–43.
3. Root M, Orien W, Weed J. Normal and abnormal function of the foot. Los Angeles (CA): Clinical Biomechanics; 1977.
4. Viegas GV. Reconstruction of hallux limitus deformity using a first metatarsal sagittal-Z osteotomy. J Foot Ankle Surg 1998;37(3):204–11 [discussion: 261–2].
5. Zammit GV, Menz HB, Munteanu SE. Structural factors associated with hallux limitus/rigidus: a systemic review of case control studies. J Orthop Sports Phys Ther 2009;39(10):733–42.
6. Gibson JN, Thomson CE. Arthrodesis or total replacement arthroplasty for hallux rigidus: a randomized control trial. Foot Ankle Int 2005;296(9):680–90.
7. Jenter M, Lipton GE, Miller F. Operative treatment for hallux valgus in children with cerebral palsy. Foot Ankle Int 1998;19(12):830–5.
8. Grimes JS, Coughlin MJ. First metatarsophalangeal joint arthrodesis as a treatment for failed hallux valgus surgery. Foot Ankle Int 2006;27(11):887–93.
9. Weil LS Jr. First metatarsophalangeal joint arthrodesis. In: Chang TJ, editor. Masters techniques in podiatric surgery: the foot and ankle. Philadelphia: Lippincott Williams & Wilkins; 2005. p. 119–28.
10. Stapleton JJ, Rodriguez RH, Jeffies LC, et al. Salvage of the first ray with concomitant septic and gouty arthritis by use of a bone block joint distraction arthrodesis and external fixation. Clin Podiatr Med Surg 2008;25:755–62.
11. Brodsky JW, Ptaszek AJ, Morris SG. Salvage first MTP arthrodesis utilizing ICBG: clinical evaluation and outcome. Foot Ankle Int 2000;21(4):290–6.

Lisfranc Arthrodesis

Panagiotis Panagakos, DPM[a],*, Krupa Patel, DPM[b],
Crystal N. Gonzalez, DPM[c]

KEYWORDS

• Lisfranc • Tarsometatarsal • Arthrodesis • Fracture • Fusion

ANATOMY

The tarsometatarsal (TMT) joint or Lisfranc joint comprises the articulation between the bases of the first, second, and third metatarsals with their respective cuneiforms and the bases of the fourth and fifth metatarsals with the distal aspect of the cuboid. The TMT joint complex is a plane-gliding type of synovial joint that is supported by a strong network of dorsal, plantar, and interosseous ligaments. The lateral tarsal artery of the dorsalis pedis provides blood supply. The deep peroneal, medial plantar, lateral plantar, and sural nerves provide nerve supply.[1]

The unique bony and ligamentous anatomy of the metatarsals, cuneiforms, and cuboid provide the architecture for the stable transverse and longitudinal arches of the foot. A cross section of the transverse arch reveals a structure similar to a Roman arch, which has inherent stability. A Roman, or centenary, arch has a central keystone that is bordered by voussoirs, or wedge-shaped bricks, that provide a locked structure. When examining the transverse arch of the foot, the second metatarsal and middle cuneiform joint act as the keystone and the wedge-shaped medial and lateral cuneiforms provide the struts that create a strong stable complex. The middle cuneiform is the smallest of the cuneiforms and is recessed approximately 8 mm relative to the medial cuneiform and 4 mm relative to the lateral cuneiform.[2] This locks the second metatarsal within the complex, adding to the stability of the joint.

A complex network of dorsal, plantar, and interosseous ligaments provides additional stability to the TMT joint. The plantar ligaments are stronger than the dorsal ligaments, which accounts for a predisposition for dorsal dislocation with injury.[3] The second metatarsal is anchored to the medial column by the strong Lisfranc ligament. The Lisfranc ligament is the strongest of the multiple ligaments within the complex measuring 1.0 cm in height and 0.5 cm in thickness.[2,3]

The authors have nothing to disclose.

[a] Foot and Ankle Care Associates, LLC, Hahnemann University Hospital, Overlook Hospital, 612 West Fingerboard Road, Staten Island, NY 10305, USA
[b] Foot and Ankle Specialists of New Jersey, 715 Central Avenue, Westfield, NJ 07090, USA
[c] Allentown Family Foot Care, PC, Lehigh Valley Health Network, St Luke's Health Network, Sacred Heart Hospital, 6690 Hauser Road, I302, Macungie, PA 18062, USA
* Corresponding author.
E-mail address: peterdpm@gmail.com

MECHANISM OF INJURY

Injuries to the TMT joint complex account for 0.2% of all fractures, with an incidence of 1 in 55,000 yearly.[4,5] Injuries are usually indirect, caused by axial loading on a plantar-flexed foot. These low-energy injuries tend to be missed because frank dislocation is not always present. Purely ligamentous injuries to the TMT joint complex are associated with longer recovery times and persistent symptoms at the area.[6] Direct injury can result from a motor vehicle accident, fall, or crush injury. These types of injuries are higher energy and, if diagnosis is missed, can result in compartment syndrome because of the close proximity of the neurovascular bundle.

CLASSIFICATIONS

Quenu and Kuss[7] were the first to classify TMT injuries in 1909. Their classification divided injuries into homolateral, isolateral, and divergent. The classification described the direction of dislocation of the metatarsals with respect to the cuneiforms and cuboid.[7] In 1982, Hardcastle and colleagues[8] elaborated on the Quenu and Kuss classification, by dividing injuries into 3 categories: A, B, and C. Type A injuries were complete displacement of all metatarsals (total incongruity) in the sagittal or transverse plane. Type B injuries were partially incongruous, and type C injuries were divergent. In 1986, Myerson and colleagues[9] further subdivided the Hardcastle classification. They described type B1 to be partially incongruous with medial dislocation with displacement of the first metatarsal in isolation or in combination with displacement of the lesser tarsus. Type B2 was partially incongruous with lateral dislocation with the first metatarsal unaffected. Type C1 was described as partially divergent with the first metatarsal displaced medially and a portion of the lateral complex displaced laterally in the sagittal and/or transverse planes. Type C2 was described as total divergent with the first metatarsal displace medially and the lateral complex displaced laterally.

DIAGNOSIS/IMAGING

The diagnosis of a Lisfranc injury can be difficult. Often, a patient presents after an injury with midfoot swelling, ecchymosis, and sometimes frank dislocation of the medial and/or lateral column (**Fig. 1**). A subtle dislocation of the TMT joint or a purely ligamentous injury to the complex is more complicated to diagnose.

The standard radiographs that need to be taken when assessing the TMT joint complex are weight-bearing dorsal plantar, medial oblique, and lateral views. We recommend that bilateral views be taken in the case of a more subtle injury. On a standard dorsal plantar radiograph, the medial border of the second metatarsal should be in line with the middle cuneiform without gapping or obliquity. The fourth metatarsal and the medial cuboid should be aligned on the oblique view. The lateral view should show continuity of the superior border of the metatarsal and the cuneiform.

Myerson and colleagues[9] described a pathognomonic sign called the fleck sign that represents an avulsion of the second metatarsal-middle cuneiform ligament. This sign is not always present when the TMT joint complex is injured but is a definite indicator of a diastasis when it is seen on radiographs. If no fleck sign is seen, radiographs should be inspected for displacement of more than 2 mm between the first and second metatarsal bases, which is indicates a Lisfranc injury.[10]

Advanced imaging is recommended when operative treatment is going to be performed or when a purely ligamentous Lisfranc injury is suspected. Computed tomography (CT) evaluation can aid in surgical planning and assessing the extent of articular

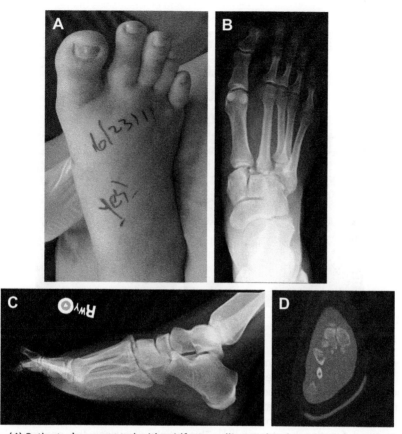

Fig. 1. (*A*) Patient who presented with midfoot swelling and ecchymosis to foot after being stepped on by a horse. (*B*) Dorsal plantar radiograph showing fleck sign and Lisfranc injury with total dislocation of TMT joint. (*C*) Lateral radiograph showing dorsal dislocation of TMT joint. (*D*) Coronal computed tomography (CT) scan showing Lisfranc fracture with dislocation and comminution of metatarsal bases 1, 2, 3 and dislocation of 4 and 5. (*E*) Three-dimensional (3D) CT reconstruction showing dislocation at TMT complex. (*Courtesy of Dr Steven Boc, DPM, FACFAS, FACFAOM, Philadelphia, PA.*)

involvement of any associated fracture. Three-dimensional (3D) reconstruction CT imaging is often performed at our facility to better visualize the disorder (see **Fig. 1**B–E). Stress radiographs are useful but difficult to perform because of patient discomfort. We routinely perform these during surgery. MR imaging is useful for subtle injuries to diagnose purely ligamentous injuries.

OPEN REDUCTION INTERNAL FIXATION INDICATIONS

Lisfranc injuries are rare, and most are unrecognized, misdiagnosed, or there is a delay in the diagnosis. They are severe injuries that, if untreated, have negative sequelae on the patient's function and overall quality of life. Myerson and colleagues[9] stated that there is no place for conservative treatment of fractures or fracture-dislocation of the Lisfranc joint. We strongly agree. Although most foot and ankle surgeons agree that surgical intervention is necessary for injuries of this complex joint structure, there

E

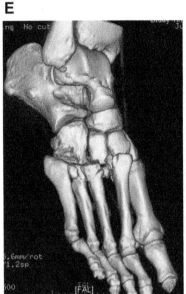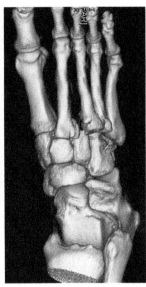

Fig. 1. (*continued*)

is controversy about how to manage it. Some investigators advocate open reduction internal fixation (ORIF), whereas others recommend performing an arthrodesis. Most of the current literature supports ORIF of Lisfranc injuries as the primary treatment. The mainstay of surgical treatment of Lisfranc injuries, which all investigators agree on, is achieving a good anatomic reduction, which has been shown to be associated with a good functional outcome.[10,11] This article discusses the controversies of surgical management of the Lisfranc joint in the literature and our indications for surgical management. Our indications for ORIF of the Lisfranc joint complex are as follows:

1. Fractures of the Lisfranc joints without extensive damage to articular cartilage
2. Extra-articular Lisfranc fractures
3. Fractures of the Lisfranc joints in athletes
4. Pediatric fractures in which there is osseous immaturity
5. Subtle Lisfranc injuries with slight displacement
6. Younger active patients in whom maintenance of motion is desired
7. Older patients with poor bone quality
8. Low-energy Lisfranc fractures

Myerson and Cerrato[10] discussed the treatment of Lisfranc fractures[10] in high-performance athletes. They concluded that primary arthrodesis is a difficult operation and the resulting stiffness may not be desirable compared with the outcome in a patient who recovers well from ORIF or closed reduction and internal fixation. Primary arthrodesis is not recommended for athletes, regardless of the potential for a rapid return to activity. They think that maintenance of motion in the medial column as well as the limited motion in the middle column is necessary to restore full function in these patients.[10] Vertullo and Nunley[13] also stated that treatment of subtle Lisfranc injuries with primary arthrodesis can be done, but is controversial in athletes. The risk of nonunion is difficult to accept, and return to professional sport after primary Lisfranc arthrodesis is rare.[12,13] We agree with all the investigators that Lisfranc arthrodesis in an athlete should be reserved only if significant chondral injury is present at the time of open reduction. A semiprofessional wrestler sustained a Lisfranc fracture-dislocation and was treated with ORIF (Fig. 2). It has been 2 years since the ORIF and the patient has returned to his normal level of activity without any pain or limitations.

We have seen good outcomes when following these indications for ORIF of the Lisfranc joints. We routinely do not remove the hardware after ORIF, even after healing is complete. There is no need for a second surgery unless there is hardware failure or pain from prominent screws. In our experience, it is rarely necessary to remove hardware after ORIF of the Lisfranc joint.

Fusion Indications

In 2006, Coetzee and Ly[14] described their selective indications for a primary fusion of the Lisfranc joints. They performed primary fusions when major ligamentous disruptions and multidirectional instability of the Lisfranc joints, comminuted intra-articular fractures at the bases of the first or second metatarsal, and crush injuries of the midfoot with an intra-articular fracture-dislocation are present. Their contraindications for primary fusion are Lisfranc injuries in children with open physis, subtle Lisfranc injuries with minimal or no displacement, unidirectional Lisfranc instability, and unstable extra-articular fractures of the metatarsal bases with unknown amounts of ligamentous disruption.[14] The investigators agree with Coetzee and Ly's[14] indications and contraindications for arthrodesis of the Lisfranc joint, but they only include the most common indications that are trauma related. Chronic pain and deformity can occur with ignored Lisfranc injuries (Fig. 3). In such cases, an arthrodesis is indicated (Fig. 4).

A controversy exists as to whether the Lisfranc joint complex should be fused primarily or reserved strictly for a salvage procedure. According to the literature, primary arthrodesis is not recommended for Lisfranc complex injuries.[15,16] Instead, arthrodesis has been reserved as a salvage procedure after failed ORIF, for a delayed or missed diagnosis, and for severely comminuted intra-articular fractures of the TMT joints.[14,16] However, in the more recent literature, a strong indication for primary arthrodesis of the TMT joints has been discussed. Granberry and colleagues[17] recommended primary fusion in any unstable injury requiring open reduction because of the high incidence of these injuries that went on to arthrodesis. Sangeorzan and colleagues[18] found a positive correlation between early arthrodesis following failed

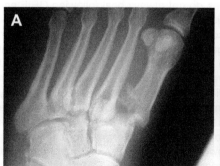
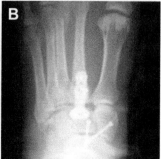

Fig. 2. (A) Preoperative Lisfranc fracture-dislocation of a semiprofessional athlete. (B) Postoperative ORIF with good anatomic reduction.

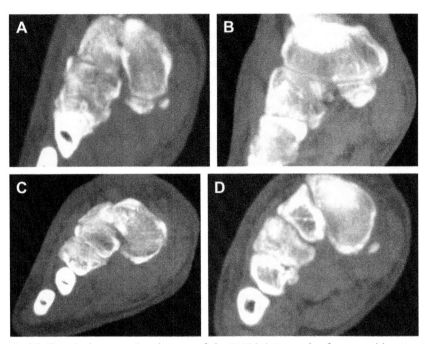

Fig. 3. (*A*) Chronic degenerative changes of the TMT joint complex from an old untreated Lisfranc injury. (*B*) Degenerative changes of the first TMT. (*C*) Degenerative changes of inter-cuneiform joints. (*D*) Degenerative changes present within the bases of third and fourth metatarsals.

primary treatment with positive results. A primary arthrodesis potentially prevents a patient from developing a painful, deformed foot and decreases or prevents the need for further surgery and further disability. Henning and colleagues[19] concluded that primary arthrodesis resulted in a statistically significant decrease in the number of follow-up surgeries performed compared with primary ORIF if hardware removal is routinely performed. Patients treated with primary arthrodesis for primarily ligamentous joint injuries function as well as those patients treated with primary ORIF.

Kuo and colleagues[20] suggested that there is a subgroup of patients with a purely ligamentous Lisfranc injury who may better treated with primary fusion. They found that purely ligamentous Lisfranc injuries do not always heal following ORIF and that there was a tendency for this type of injury to result in osteoarthritis.[14,20] In 2006, Coetzee and Ly[14] published their results comparing ORIF and primary arthrodesis of the Lisfranc joint consisting of purely ligamentous injuries. They enrolled 41 patients with an isolated acute or subacute primary ligamentous Lisfranc joint injury in a prospective randomized study. Twenty patients were treated with ORIF and 21 with primary arthrodesis of the medial 2 or 3 rays. At 2 years after surgery, the mean American Orthopaedic Foot and Ankle Society (AOFAS) midfoot score was 68.6 in the ORIF group and 88 points in the arthrodesis group. Of the 20 patients in the ORIF group, 16 underwent a secondary surgery to remove prominent or painful hardware. Follow-up radiographs showed evidence of loss of correction, increasing deformity, and degenerative joint disease in 15 patients. Five of these patients in the ORIF group had persistent pain and developed osteoarthritis, and were eventually treated with arthrodesis. The patients in the arthrodesis group stated that their

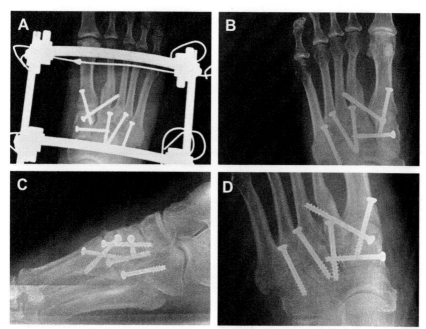

Fig. 4. (*A*) Immediate postoperative radiograph of Lisfranc fusion with external fixation. (*B*) Complete fusion of the TMT complex. (*C*) Lateral radiograph showing complete fusion of TMT complex. (*D*) Complete TMT fusion. (*Courtesy of* Dr Steven Boc, DPM, FACFAS, FAC-FAOM, Philadelphia, PA.)

postoperative level of activity was 92% of their preinjury level compared with only 65% for the patients who had ORIF. Coetzee and Ly[14] study concluded that primary stable arthrodesis of the Lisfranc joint complex has a better short-term and medium-term outcome than ORIF. Kuo and colleagues[20] found that the mean AOFAS score for mid-foot ORIF was 78.8 compared with the 57.1 found by Coetzee and Ly,[14] but Coetzee and Ly's[14] mean AOFAS score for their arthrodesis group was higher at 86.9 points. They concluded that, in primarily ligamentous injuries, healing of the ligaments and capsules provided insufficient strength to maintain the initial reduction.[14]

The authors think that designating treatment of a Lisfranc injury for arthrodesis or ORIF is patient specific, with factors such as age, physical activity, bone density quality, timing of the diagnosis, amount of deformity, or presence of osteoarthritis playing important roles that are not discussed by the investigators of these various studies. We have seen great results with both our ORIF and arthrodesis patients. Our indications for arthrodesis of the Lisfranc joint complex are as follows:

1. Severe fractures of the joint complex that involve the articular cartilage
2. Any disorder that causes cystic bone changes within 1 or any of the Lisfranc joints (eg, benign bone tumor; **Fig. 5**)
3. Failed previous ORIF of any Lisfranc injury with persistent pain
4. Chronic ignored or misdiagnosed Lisfranc injuries that have led to severe degenerative joint disease
5. Any joint complex with severe atraumatic osteoarthritis
6. Any joint complex with severe deformity in any cardinal plane
7. Persistent pain and disability

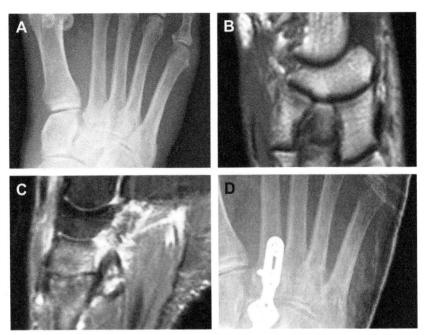

Fig. 5. (*A*) Osteochondroma affecting the second TMT joint. (*B*) Magnetic resonance imaging (MRI) showing enchondroma of second TMT joint. (*C*) Fat-suppression MRI showing enchondroma of the second TMT joint. (*D*) Arthrodesis of second TMT for alleviation of pain secondary to benign bone tumor.

Following these indications, we have seen good to excellent results for patients returning to function, and improved pain levels. After osseous union has been achieved radiographically and patients are able to ambulate in normal shoe gear, they are casted for accommodative orthotics.

There is an emerging technique that might replace primary arthrodesis of the Lisfranc joint complex for purely ligamentous injuries. Neoligamentoplasty of the TMT joints, described by Nery and colleagues[21] from Brazil, is showing promising results. They resect the torn ligaments, anatomically reduce the subluxed joints, and then isometrically reconstruct the ligaments of the TMT joint. In their study with a mean of an 8-year follow-up, 17 patients (85%) had excellent or good results, whereas 3 (15%) had fair or poor results. This new technique has not yet been attempted by the authors. In the near future, a randomized prospective study should be done comparing primary arthrodesis with neoligamentoplasty for the treatment of purely ligamentous Lisfranc injuries.

PARTIAL VERSUS COMPLETE LISFRANC ARTHRODESIS

Another controversy with surgical management of the Lisfranc joint when performing an arthrodesis is whether to fuse the whole complex or just the medial rays. This problem has been described in the most current literature. Mulier and colleagues[22] compared ORIF with complete arthrodesis and partial arthrodesis. They concluded that a complete fusion of all 5 TMT joints yields poor results and that ORIF provides a better functional outcome. Komeda and colleagues[23] showed that, although patients had radiographic evidence of osteoarthritis of the fourth and fifth metatarsocuboid joints, they had no pain in this location before or after surgery. They stated that the reason for this is not well understood. They found that the lateral column, which has the most motion (mean of 10°), in the sagittal plane was the least painful; however, the second TMT, which has the least motion (mean of 0.6°), was the most painful. They recommended that the lateral column not be included in the arthrodesis because the motion of the lateral column is important for optimum function.[23]

Park and colleagues[24] stated that lateral column fusion is indicated when there is degenerative arthritis limited to the lateral TMT joint, usually after trauma. There are possible detrimental biomechanical effects of having no motion at the fourth and fifth metatarsal cuboid joints. It may decrease the ability of the foot to act as a mobile adapter during the contact period of gait because there are effectively fewer bony segments in the foot to provide skeletal mobility. The procedure also increases the ground reactive forces of the fourth and fifth metatarsal heads, which could lead to metatarsalgia. One advantage of fusing the lateral column is the improved functional efficiency of the peroneus brevis, because it no longer needs to stabilize the fifth metatarsal posteriorly against the cuboid during midstance and early propulsion.[25]

Mulier and colleagues[22] compared ORIF with complete arthrodesis and partial arthrodesis in 28 patients. They found that Baltimore Painful foot Score (PFS) was higher in the ORIF group than in the complete arthrodesis group, meaning that the ORIF group had less pain. No difference in the PFS was found between the ORIF group and the partial arthrodesis group. They also noted that complications were also slightly lower in the ORIF group. They concluded that a complete arthrodesis of the Lisfranc joints should be reserved solely as a salvage procedure.

Coetzee and Ly[14] agreed with Komeda and colleagues[23] and Mulier and colleagues,[22] and proposed only fusing the medial 2 or 3 rays because it is beneficial for a patient to have motion in the lateral 2 rays and because it is not necessary to perform a complete fusion to obtain optimum results. We have performed both partial and complete arthrodesis of the Lisfranc joint complex. In our experience, there are insignificant differences after surgery in the patients' pain level or return to normal function between the 2 groups (**Fig. 6**A–C). We agree with Treadwell and Khan,[26] who stated that there was no correlation between the number of joints fused and the functional outcome. We regularly cast patients for accommodative orthotics when they are ready to return to normal function and, if necessary, tell them to wear a stiff-soled shoe. In our opinion, the custom-molded orthotics help to prevent or treat fourth or fifth ray disorders that might occur secondary to a complete arthrodesis of the Lisfranc joint complex. The use of orthotics to prevent or alleviate pain after arthrodesis is not discussed in the literature.

Fixation Techniques

The treatment of Lisfranc fracture-dislocations varies from nonsurgical treatment with closed reduction through closed reduction and percutaneous pinning, ORIF with screws, and fixation with screws combined with external fixation. For arthrodesis of the TMT joint complex, the authors advocate using interfragmentary screws with or without combination of external fixation (**Fig. 7**). Interfragmentary screws are strong and provide good compression across all joints, and external fixation provides additional stability to the fusion site by preventing shearing forces and adding additional compression across the fusion site. Buttress and locking plates can also be used in certain conditions, such as isolated joint fusions with or without bone grafting, injuries requiring deformity correction, osteopenic bone, or for Charcot midfoot reconstructive fusions. Staples can be used as adjunct fixation with plates and/or screws. The use of

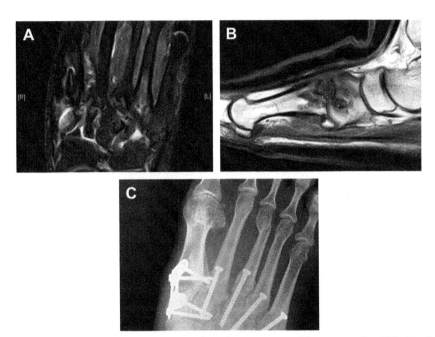

Fig. 6. (*A*) Preoperative MRI indicating Lisfranc ligament tear. (*B*) Preoperative MRI showing the extent of articular damage and deformity of Lisfranc injury. (*C*) Healed complete TMT fusion.

Kirschner wires is not recommended for arthrodesis of the Lisfranc joint complex, but they are useful for provisional fixation in maintaining proper alignment.

Screws should be used for fusion and should be large enough to provide sufficient stability. Fully threaded 3.5-mm screws inserted via lag technique or 4.0-mm partially threaded screws are appropriate for Lisfranc fusion. We prefer the using 4.0-mm partially threaded cannulated screws because of their simplicity and the ability for the guide wires to act as provisional fixation. Zonno and Myerson[27] warn not to split

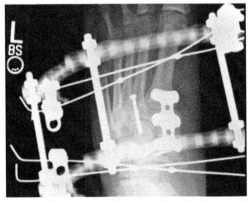

Fig. 7. Combination of internal fixation and external fixation for partial Lisfranc arthrodesis. (*Courtesy of* Dr Steven Boc, DPM, FACFAS, FACFAOM, Philadelphia, PA.)

the metatarsal bases with the last few turns of screw insertion. They advise using a burr to create a recess for the head of the screw to prevent this for the first metatarsocuneiform joint and using custom plates for the second and third metatarsocuneiform joints.[27] We have not experienced this with our patients, and regularly use screws to fuse across the Lisfranc joint complex without encountering this issue.

Coetzee and Ly[14] state that it is difficult to achieve good compression with a screw across the third TMT because of the angle required to insert the screw. They propose using a staple to fuse this joint because of its ease of insertion.[14] Kilmartin and O'Kane[28] described a fixation technique for isolated second metatarsal cuneiform joint fusion with bone graft. They prefer to use a 3-hole 2.7-mm tubular plate with cortical screws placed on either side of the joint to a single 4.0 screw. They stated that the surface area of the joint is small and passing a single 4.0 screw across it leaves little bone surface through which to achieve solid fusion.[28] In 2009, Smith and colleagues[29] described their technique for isolated arthrodesis of the second metatarsocuneiform joint. They fashioned two 0.045 K-wires into staples and inserted the arms of the staples, angulated in a divergent orientation, to achieve slight compression across the fusion site. Staples are an easy alternative for fixation but the older staples do not provide stable compression. We use them in combination with screws or plates or solely when an external fixator will be applied as well.

Mann and colleagues[30] stated that the best form of fixation involves interfragmentary screws or a medial plate, or both. No specific screw construct was noted to be better than another for the repair/fusion of multiple joints. They also recommended a buttress plate be used on the medial side of the foot when a severe abduction deformity is being corrected.

External fixation is widely used to treat fractures and limb deformities as well as its many other indications. We highly recommend the use of external fixation for arthrodesis of the Lisfranc joint complex with or without internal fixation. Untreated Lisfranc fracture commonly results in valgus malunion, which leads to shortening of the lateral column, stress on the medial column, dysfunction of the posterior tibial muscle, and flatfoot deformity. Varus malunion rarely develops from Lisfranc fracture. External fixation can allow for lengthening of the lateral and medial columns. According to Hamilton and Ford,[31] the ideal external fixator is easy to apply, lightweight, versatile, inexpensive, compatible with wound care and normal function, and rigid enough to promote healing without loss of function. External fixation can be used for primary arthrodesis, salvage arthrodesis after failed ORIF with or without angular and shortening deformities. The fusion site must be protected from shear, torsional, and bending forces.

Yamagishi and Yoshimura[32] showed that excessive shear forces promote the formation of pseudoarthrosis. A fusion site held rigidly relies increasingly on primary bone healing. If longitudinal instability exists, then the fixator must provide rigid axial stabilization.[33] The rigidity of the fixator increases when bone-to-bar distance decreases and when interpin distance decreases.[31] Choice of fixator depends largely on the surgeon's preference and training. In Hahnemann University Hospital, the external fixator of choice for Lisfranc fusion is 2 half rings connected by 3 rods (**Fig. 8**). One half ring is proximal, the other half ring is distal to the fusion sites, and the olive wires are tensioned appropriately. This construct possesses all of the qualities and advantages that are mentioned by Hamilton and Ford.[31] It is easily applied with decreased operative time compared with a traditional Ilizarov fixator. We have used this construct for midfoot fusions in combination with internal fixation. We have seen excellent results in our midfoot fusions with no signs of nonunion, probably because of the increased rigidity, stability, and compression provided by the frame. A prospective randomized study should be designed to evaluate this specific construct

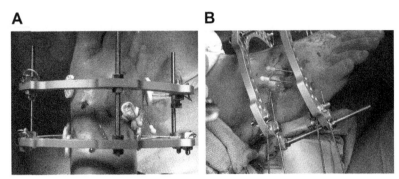

Fig. 8. (*A*) External fixation structure for Lisfranc arthrodesis. (*B*) Lateral view of midfoot fusion external fixation structure. (*Courtesy of* Dr Steven Boc, DPM, FACFAS, FACFAOM, Philadelphia, PA.)

used alone in Lisfranc fusions compared with using it in combination with internal fixation.

TECHNIQUE

In the literature in recent years there has been a standardization of operative technique, especially for incision placement for fixing Lisfranc fractures and dislocations. Many investigators have seen many preventable complications secondary to poor incision placement including, but not limited to, sensory deficit or nerve entrapments when trying to expose too many metatarsals with the incision. In addition, painful scars can result, especially when there is too much tension on the skin or the incisions are made against resting skin tension lines. The literature typically points to 3 incisional approaches that create access to the metatarsals to fixate the Lisfranc fracture. The 3 incisions to use include the medial aspect of the foot at the base of the first metatarsal extending over the medial cuneiform. This incision exposes the extensor hallucis brevis muscle. Deep to this muscle is the neurovascular bundle. Anatomy should be kept in mind when performing the dissection to avoid unnecessary dissection of the neurovascular bundles. The second incision should be over the base of the second metatarsal and should extend over the intermediate cuneiform to the distal lateral aspect of the cuneiform. This incision provides access to the second and third metatarsals and their respective cuneiforms. The last incision should be made at the base of the fourth metatarsal and extended into the cuboid. This incision creates access to the fourth and fifth metatarsals. On dissection, care must be taken with the deep peroneal, intermediate dorsal cutaneous, and medial dorsal cutaneous nerves. Aggressive dissection of the soft tissues surrounding these areas could put the nerves at risk. The lateral incision may not be necessary if there is no fracture-dislocation of the fourth and fifth metatarsal. However, if it is seen during surgery that these do need to be corrected, this lateral incision will provide adequate exposure.[34,35]

Once the base of the first metatarsal and the medial cuneiform have been exposed, the joint should be prepared. Whether the procedure is an ORIF or fusion, bone fragments and damaged cartilage need to be removed from the joint. If a fusion is being performed, then any plantar prominences need to be resected to ensure that a malunion does not occur. To help with the reduction of the deformity, the windlass mechanism should be performed to reduce the deformity. This mechanism helps to compress the joint as well as avoiding a malunion in a dorsiflexed position. Using a bone reduction clamp allows the reduction to be maintained as well as more permanent fixation to be created without loss of reduction.

When performing an ORIF, screw placement is essential for anatomic reduction, which is the goal of surgery, and maintaining anatomic reduction helps delay the development of posttraumatic arthritis. If using K-wires, it is recommended that a 0.062 K-wire be used because smaller K-wires may make it more difficult to maintain the reduction. The first K-wire should be in the orientation from plantar medial to dorsal lateral from the medial cuneiform to the base of the second metatarsal. The second K-wire should be from dorsal distal to plantar proximal, from the base of the second metatarsal to the intermediate cuneiform. The third K-wire should be dorsal distal to plantar proximal as well from the base of the first metatarsal to the medial cuneiform. The fourth K-wire should be from distal lateral to proximal medial from the base of the fifth metatarsal to the cuboid. The fifth K-wire should also be distal lateral to proximal medial from the base of the fourth metatarsal into the lateral cuneiform. An optional K-wire can be from distal dorsal to plantar proximal from the base of the third metatarsal to the lateral cuneiform. These K-wires can be used as guide wires for a 3.5 or 4.0 cannulated screw system. However, the use of screws in the fourth and fifth metatarsal is not recommended because of their independent ranges of motion. The fourth and fifth metatarsals usually move back into place with reduction of the third metatarsal.[36]

When closing the layers in the foot, special attention should be paid to closing the periosteum and the joint capsule, which provides blood supply to the healing fractures and aids in the healing. However, closure of the subcutaneous tissue should be avoided. Entrapment of the nerves in this layer poses a risk when trying to close these layers.[37]

POSTOPERATIVE CARE

After surgery, patients need to be non–weight bearing for 8 to 10 weeks. Many studies have shown that patients who bore weight on their feet before 6 weeks had an increased incidence of disability.[33] The patient should remain in a Jones compression-type splint to help with the reduction of edema into the foot. At 2 weeks, the stitches or staples should be removed. For the next 4 to 6 weeks, a below-knee cast should be used to maintain strict non–weight bearing. The 6-week to 8-week mark is when the K-wires, if used, should be removed. Also at this time, if an external fixation device is used, with confirmation of adequate bone healing on radiograph, the external fixation device should be removed. Patients should begin guarded toe-touch weight bearing at home with the assistance of a CAM (controlled ankle movement) walker. At the 8-week to 10-week mark, as long as the radiographs show adequate joint healing and/or fusion, depending on what technique is used, the patient may begin to weight bear fully in a sneaker. The patient may need physical therapy to recondition the muscles. Orthotics may be discussed at this point because the swelling should be decreased and an adequate cast of the foot can be performed.

COMPLICATIONS

Although postoperative complications are inevitable, recognition of the complication is imperative to determine the postoperative outcome. Preoperative planning is important to help prevent complications. The usual course of fractures and dislocations is to have some swelling before the surgery. Applying a Jones compressive dressing before surgery helps to manage the edema. The foot should be examined every 2 to 3 days to determine when there is adequate reduction of swelling to perform surgery. If surgery is performed before swelling resolves, there is the risk of wound dehiscence and damage to the soft tissues.

Posttraumatic arthritis is a well-known complication of Lisfranc injuries. Current literature suggests that the incidence of arthritis is as high as 60% to 80%. Many investigators state that arthritis will probably occur and that the patient should be informed that it will probably not be prevented. Arthritis has a variety of clinical presentation clinically and radiographically.[36] Infection, hematoma, deep vein thrombosis, pulmonary embolism, and wound dehiscence are the initial postoperative complications that need to kept in mind. During the non–weight-bearing period, osteopenia and atrophy should be monitored on physical examination and on radiograph evaluation. If K-wires are used, pin tract infections as well as movement of the wires need to be kept in mind. If the wires move, then loss of the reduction must be considered. Long-term side effects include arthritic changes, delayed or malunion, chronic pain, swelling, and reflex sympathetic dystrophy.

DISCUSSION

Lisfranc fracture-dislocation is an uncommon injury. It accounts for only for 0.2% of fractures every year. However, it is one of the most misdiagnosed injuries because it can occur subtly. If not recognized early, many patients will experience arthritic changes in later years. A good understanding of the anatomy is the key to recognizing the fracture and dislocation.

Selection of procedure, whether ORIF or arthrodesis, depends on the foot and ankle surgeon's preference. Some patients may not agree with a primary fusion but they must understand that there can be a high rate of arthritic changes even with the most perfect ORIF. Choice of fixation can be from simple K-wires, screws, and plates to external fixation. Surgeons should choose the method of fixation with which they are most comfortable.

After surgery, the patient should remain non–weight bearing for at least 6 to 8 weeks or until adequate healing is noted on radiograph. If weight bearing is rushed, there is a high risk for malalignment of the bones. Patients should be monitored closely for complications and patients should be aware that arthritic changes are almost guaranteed.

Lisfranc fracture-dislocations are complex fractures that need to be identified early to prevent complications. They should be reapproximated whether the joint is open reduced with internal fixation or fused.

REFERENCES

1. Agur AM, Dalley AF. Lower limb. In: Grant's atlas of anatomy. 11th edition. USA: Lippincott Williams & Wilkins; 2005. p. 504–662.
2. Serragian SK. Syndesmology. In: Serrafian SK, editor. Anatomy of the foot and ankle: descriptive, topographic, functional. 2nd edition. USA: Lippincott Company; 1993. p. 159–217.
3. Kura H, Luo ZP, Kitaoka HB, et al. Mechanical behavior of the Lisfranc and dorsal cuneometatarsal ligaments: in vitro biomechanical study. J Orthop Trauma 2001; 15(2):101–10.
4. Aitken AP, Poulson D. Dislocation of the tarsometatarsal joint. J Bone Joint Surg Am 1963;45:246–60.
5. English TA. Dislocations of the metatarsal bone and adjacent toe. J Bone Joint Surg Br 1964;46:700–4.

6. Richter M, Wippermann B, Krettek C. Fractures and fracture dislocations of the midfoot: occurrence, causes and long-term results. Foot Ankle Int 2001; 22:392–8.

7. Quenu E, Kuss G. Etude sur les luxations du metatarse (luxations metatarsotarsiennes) du diastasis entre le 1er et le 2e metatarsien. Rev Chir 1909;39:281–336, 720–91, 1093–134.

8. Hardcastle PH, Reschauer R, Kutscha-Lissber E, et al. Injuries to the tarsometatarsal joint. Incidence, classification and treatment. J Bone Joint Surg Br 1982;64: 349–56.

9. Myerson MS, Fisher RT, Burgess AR, et al. Fracture dislocations of the tarsometatarsal joints: end results correlated with pathology and treatment. Foot Ankle 1986;9:225–42.

10. Myerson MS, Cerrato RA. Current management of tarsometatarsal injuries in the athlete. J Bone Joint Surg Am 2008;90:2522–33.

11. Desmond EA, Chou LB. Current concepts review: Lisfranc injuries. Foot Ankle Int 2006;27(8):653–60.

12. Ardoin TG, Anderson RB. Subtle Lisfranc injury. Techniques in Foot & Ankle Surgery 2010;9:100–6.

13. Vertullo CJ, Nunley MD. Participation in sports after arthrodesis of the foot and ankle. Foot Ankle Int 2002;7:625–8.

14. Coetzee CJ, Ly TV. Treatment of primarily ligamentous Lisfranc joint injuries: primary arthrodesis compared with open reduction and internal fixation. Surgical technique. J Bone Joint Surg Am 2007;89:122–7.

15. Lenczner EM, Waddell JP, Graham JD. Tarsal-metatarsal (Lisfranc) dislocation. J Trauma 1974;14:1012–20.

16. Arntz CT, Veith RG, Hansen ST Jr. Fractures and fracture-dislocations of the tarsometatarsal joint. J Bone Joint Surg Am 1988;70:173–81.

17. Granberry W, Lipscomb P. Dislocation of the tarsometatarsal joints. Surg Gynecol Obstet 1962;114:467–9.

18. Sangeorzan B, Veith R, Hansen S. Salvage of the Lisfranc's tarsometatarsal joint by arthrodesis. Foot Ankle Int 1990;10:193–200.

19. Henning JA, Jones CB, Sietsema D, et al. Open reduction internal fixation versus primary arthrodesis for Lisfranc Injuries: a prospective randomized study. Foot Ankle Int 2009;30(10):913–22.

20. Kuo RS, Tejwani NC, Digiovanni CW, et al. Outcome after open reduction internal fixation of Lisfranc joint injuries. J Bone Joint Surg Am 2000;82:1609–18.

21. Nery C, Ressio C, Alloza JF. Neoligamentoplasty for the treatment of subtle ligament lesions of the intercuneiform and tarsometatarsal joints. Tech Foot Ankle 2010;9:92–9.

22. Mulier T, Reynders P, Dereymaeker G, et al. Severe Lisfranc injuries: primary arthrodesis or ORIF? Foot Ankle Int 2002;23(10):902–5.

23. Komeda GA, Myerson MS, Biddinger KR. Results of arthrodesis of the tarsometatarsal joints after traumatic injury. J Bone Joint Surg Am 1996;78:1665–76.

24. Park DS, Schram AJ, Stone NM. Isolated lateral tarsometatarsal joint arthrodesis: a case report. J Foot Ankle Surg 2000;39(4):239–43.

25. Root ML, Orien WP, Weed JH. Normal and abnormal function of the foot, vol. 2. Los Angeles (CA): Clinical Biomechanics; 1977.

26. Treadwell JR, Khan MD. Lisfranc arthrodesis for chronic pain: a cannulated screw technique. J Foot Ankle Surg 1998;37:28–36.

27. Zonno AJ, Myerson MS. Surgical correction of midfoot arthritis with and without deformity. Foot Ankle Clin 2011;16:35–47.

28. Kilmartin TE, O'Kane C. Fusion of the second metatarsocuneiform joint for the painful osteoarthrosis. Foot Ankle Int 2008;29(11):1079–87.
29. Smith SE, Camasta CA, Cass AD. A technique for isolated arthrodesis of the second metatarsocuneiform joint. J Foot Ankle Surg 2009;48(5):606–11.
30. Mann RA, Prieskorn D, Sobel M. Mid-tarsal and tarsometatarsal arthrodesis for primary degenerative osteoarthrosis or osteoarthrosis after trauma. J Bone Joint Surg Am 1996;78:1376–85.
31. Hamilton GA, Ford LA. External fixation of the foot and ankle elective indications and techniques for external fixation in the midfoot. Clin Podiatr Med Surg 2003; 20:45–63.
32. Yamagishi M, Yoshimura Y. he biomechanics of fracture healing. J Bone Joint Surg Am 1955;37(5):1035–68.
33. Kenwright J, Goodship AE. Controlled mechanical stimulation in the treatment of tibial fractures. Clin Orthop 1989;241:36–47.
34. Sands AK. Open reduction and internal fixation of Lisfranc/tarsometatarsal injuries. In: Foot and ankle surgery. 1st edition. USA: Saunders Elsevier; 2010. p. 246–56.
35. Caldarella DJ. Surgery of the Lisfranc joint. In: Master techniques in podiatric surgery: the foot and ankle. 1st edition. USA: Lippincott Williams & Wilkins; 2005. p. 189–210.
36. Douglas SA. Lisfranc and midfoot fractures. In: Fractures of the foot and ankle. 1st edition. USA: ElSevier Saunders; 2004. p. 95–149.
37. Easley ME. Midfoot arthrodesis. In: Operative techniques in foot and ankle surgery. 1st edition. USA: Lippincott Williams & Wilkins; 2011. p. 286–307.

Subtalar Joint Arthrodesis

Ramon Lopez, DPM[a,b], Tarika Singh, DPM, AACFAS[c],
Samantha Banga, DPM[a],*, Nafisa Hasan, DPM[a]

KEYWORDS

- Subtalar joint • Arthrodesis • Biomechanics
- Rearfoot correction

Isolated subtalar joint arthrodesis has gained popularity more recently. In the past, isolated talocalcaneal fusions were rarely done because it was considered to have undesirable arthritic effects on surrounding joints. After Astion and colleagues simulated isolated arthrodesis of the subtalar joint, they found that more than half of calcaneocuboid joint motion is retained. About 26% of the talonavicular joint motion and 46% of the posterior tibial tendon excursion was retained.[1] Although it was not favored, research has shown that it preserved rearfoot motion, did not increase the risk of arthritis in adjacent joints, and is a less complex operative procedure. It decreases the chance of midtarsal joint nonunion and malunion postoperatively.[2]

This article takes an in-depth approach to isolated talocalcaneal fusions. Anatomy and biomechanics of the subtalar joint are reviewed. Clinical presentation and radiologic evaluation are discussed. Lastly, conservative treatment, operative technique, and postoperative management are outlined.

ANATOMY

When doing a subatalar arthrodesis, it is important to understand the anatomy in the subtalar joint in order to preserve soft tissue and maintain the blood supply of the talus and calcaneus without further damage. The subtalar joint consists of 3 facets on the dorsal surface of the calcaneus and plantar surface of the talus. The facets are the anterior, middle, and posterior. The anterior and middle facets are convex in nature whereas the posterior facet is generally concave in nature.[3]

This arthrodesis can be performed arthroscopically by using anterolateral and posterolateral portals. The posterolateral portal is located just lateral to the Achilles tendon. The anterolateral portal is identified as 1 cm distal and 0.5 cm anterior to

[a] Hahnemann University Hospital, Drexel University College of Medicine; Philadelphia, PA, USA
[b] Hosham Foot and Ankle Group, Horsham, PA, USA
[c] The Foot and Ankle Group, P.C. Aria Health, Philadelphia, PA, USA
* Corresponding author.
E-mail address: Samantha_banga@yahoo.com

Clin Podiatr Med Surg 29 (2012) 67–75
doi:10.1016/j.cpm.2011.09.003   **podiatric.theclinics.com**
0891-8422/12/$ – see front matter © 2012 Elsevier Inc. All rights reserved.

the tip of the lateral malleolus. A posteromedial portal may be used, but caution must be taken to identify and avoid the tibial nerve and the posterior tibial artery. An accessory portal can be made through the sinus tarsi.[4]

The plantar surface of the body of the talus consists of the posterior calcaneal articular facet, which runs anterolaterally and is concave in nature. This facet articulates with the dorsal surface of the calcaneus known as the posterior talar articular surface. This surface also runs anterolaterally and is convex in nature.[5]

Anterior to the posterior talar articular surface lies a groove named the sulcus calcanei. It joins the sulcus tali, a groove on the talus, to become the canalis tarsi and sinus tarsi. The interosseus talocalcaneal ligament is located within this canal. It is important to try to preserve this ligament, as it does carry some blood supply to the area. Other ligaments such as the bifurcate ligament, the cervical ligament, and the stem of the inferior extensor retinaculum also can be found in this region. They all attach laterally to sulcus calcanei.

The blood supply to the area of the subtalar joint comes from the artery of the sinus tarsi, a branch of the lateral tarsal artery, and the artery of the canalis tarsi, a branch of the posterior tibial artery. The medial side of the body of the talus receives the blood supply from deltoid branches of the canalis tarsi. It is important to preserve the blood supply, as disruption could cause aseptic necrosis.

BIOMECHANICS

The subtalar joint is a prominent joint in the foot in that it dictates the movements of the midtarsal joint as well as the forefoot. The 3 articulations between the talus and calcaneus, namely the anterior, middle, and posterior facets, move in unison during motion.[6] The movements of these articulations are stabilized by ligaments; if any damage occurs to the ligaments the result is abnormal motion at the joint. The joint itself allows for transmission of rotation from the leg and ankle to the distal articulations of the foot, as well as providing for shock absorption during the early part of the stance phase.[7,8]

Much controversy exists as to the type of motion that occurs at the subtalar joint. Some[9] claim a sliding type motion, whereas others such as Hicks[10] describe rotational motion. In recent literature the motion is described more as a screwlike motion with multiaxial motion involving rotations and translations.[11] Many experiments have been performed using loading configurations to deduce the motion at the joint. Hicks[10] maintained that the joint motion was the same whether the foot was loaded or unloaded. Leardini and colleagues[12] deduced that subtalar motion occurs when external deviations are applied, but was recovered as soon as the deviations were removed.

The axis of the subtalar joint is another subject of debate. As the joint is put through motion the axis changes its orientation because it is likely that the joint is not fully congruous throughout that motion. Given that the subtalar joint is a diarthrodial joint, Shephard[13] described the axis of joint rotation to run from anteromediosuperior to posterolateroinferior, passing through the tuberosity of the calcaneus upwards and slightly medial to the neck of the talus forward, crossing the canalis tarsi.

PATHOLOGY AND INDICATIONS

Pathology that leads to degeneration of the subtalar joint and chronic pain may require subtalar joint arthrodesis. Pain and deformity are the most important indications that would lead to isolated subtalar fusion. Rearfoot varus or valgus can be corrected during talocalcaneal fusion.

Posttraumatic arthritis may result from calcaneal or talar fractures, whether the fracture was originally treated conservatively or surgically. Primary talocalcaneal arthritis can also be treated with a fusion. Residual congenital deformities including talipes equinovarus, talocalcaneal coalitions, and calcaneovalgus can eventually lead to arthritis of the subtalar joint. Posterior tibial tendon dysfunction may also lead to a symptomatic subtalar joint.[2]

The surgeon may opt to primarily fuse an intra-articular comminuted calcaneal fracture. Cartilage damage and inability to reconstruct the posterior facet following a severely comminuted fracture often leads to severe discomfort, decreased quality of life, inability to perform activities of daily living, and the need for eventual subtalar joint arthrodesis. Therefore, the surgeon may opt to save the patient future discomfort and primarily fuse if initial surgical management is chosen. Initial nonsurgical management is often chosen if there is minimal hindfoot deformity followed by subsequent subtalar arthrodesis.

CONSERVATIVE TREATMENT

Conservative treatment is the first-line treatment for subtalar joint pain and arthritis. Oral nonsteroidal anti-inflammatories are often attempted first. Sinus tarsi/subtalar joint injections consisting of a mixture of local anesthetic and steroids are helpful in temporarily relieving arthritis pain and inflammation. Bracing and physical therapy are other conservative treatments. When activities of daily living are affected by chronic subtalar joint pain, patients then opt for surgical treatment. Surgeons may attempt arthroscopic treatment before resorting to subtalar joint fusion.

CLINICAL SIGNS AND SYMPTOMS

The clinical signs and symptoms of subtalar joint pain are different depending on the etiology. Patients will often complain of pain in the hindfoot and ankle. The nature of the pain is often described as dull and stiff. These individuals will often present with a valgus or varus deformity of the hindfoot. On occasion, a patient may describe the pain as numbness depending on the etiology of the subtalar joint pain.

In addition, a surgeon may also notice swelling of the ankle joints as well as swelling in the entire hindfoot. If there is a history of intra-articular calcaneal fractures, one may notice a decrease in the heel height as well as a widened heel. These patients will often complain of discomfort and difficulty in wearing their shoes. Patients will complain of the pain worsening throughout the day because of this discomfort.

On clinical evaluation, the surgeon may or may not find restriction on range of motion of the ankle joint. Patients with restricted range of motion will often complain of their ankles/foot locking and difficulty walking. In addition, these individuals will complain of muscular pain on the back of their leg and difficulty walking. Therefore, depending on the origin of the subtalar joint pain, its presentation can be very diverse.

PHYSICAL EXAMINATION

When seen acutely, patients with subtalar joint pain/instability may have what appears to be a severe ankle sprain. On examination they present with lateral ecchymosis, edema, and tenderness. Such patients may also have a great amount of inversion when stress is applied to the ankle. On closer examination one may note lateral swelling that is associated with subtalar joint tenderness. More often, patients with subtalar joint pain/instability present later with vague complaints of pain and discomfort and a history of chronic injury to the area; they also may have ankle and hindfoot stiffness associated with disuse.[14] Therefore, it is imperative that the physical examination include multiple factors: amount of pain on palpation, gait evaluation, and range of motion as well as quality of motion. Examination should also include evaluation of the ipsilateral side.

Subtalar joint motion is assessed with the patient in a prone position. The heel is bisected and is compared with the lower leg as the calcaneus is inverted and everted. Normal range of motion is a 2:1 (20°–10°) relationship of inversion to eversion. While maneuvering the calcaneus one should evaluate the quality of motion by feeling for any crepitus (a grating-type feeling).

Thermann and colleagues[15] described an examination maneuver to support a theory of rotational component in addition to tilt in subtalar joint instability. The test is described as holding the foot in 10° of dorsiflexion as the heel and foot are held rigid while an inversion and internal rotation stress is applied to the heel. An adduction stress is then applied to the forefoot. While performing this maneuver the examiner felt a medial shift of the calcaneus under the talus.[15]

Subtalar pain and instability is a complex condition with many elements. It is crucial to have a thorough physical examination as a baseline before proceeding with any treatment. Physical examination can be useful in correlation with diagnostic imaging.

RADIOGRAPHIC FINDINGS

When evaluating the subtalar joint it is typical to obtain weight-bearing anteroposterior, lateral, and medial oblique views. The radiograph will show joint arthrosis, which includes nonuniform joint space narrowing, subchondral sclerosis, and osteophyte formation. A calcaneal axial view is often also obtained to evaluate hindfoot position as well as for tarsal coalitions. It is recommended to obtain views of the unaffected side and to compare these with the injured side (**Fig. 1**).

Evaluation of a lateral-view radiograph in a normal foot reveals the sinus tarsi at approximately the level of the neck of the talus. The sinus tarsi size wise is moderate, neither too prominent nor nonexistent. The posterior facets of the calcaneus and talus are congruent, and the posterior facet of the calcaneus bears the majority of compressive forces originating from body weight.[16]

In subtalar joint pronation evaluation, of the lateral radiograph reveals the talus in a more anterior position when compared with the rectus foot. In pronation the position of the talus shifts to a more plantar medial direction, and while this is occurring the calcaneus everts. In a very severely pronated foot the sinus tarsi may be hard to visualize at all. As the talus moves anterior in severe pronation, the talar posterior process

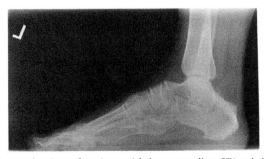

Fig. 1. Pre operative evaluation of patient with long standing STJ pain/instability.

articulates with the calcaneal posterior facet. This misalignment eventually leads to degenerative changes.

While evaluating both lateral and dorsoplantar radiographs, it is possible to visualize a cyma line. The cyma line is S-shaped and runs through the calcaneal cuboid and talonavicular joints. The continuity of the line is disrupted in pronation, in that one sees an anterior break in the line on lateral radiographic examination. The break in the cyma line is more posterior in excessive supination.[17]

In subtalar joint supination the talus moves posteriorly and abducts. The posterior facet of the talus moves posterior on the calcaneus and the sinus tarsi appears to be greatly increased in size. Again, the misalignment of the joint will lead to eventual degeneration of the joint and will appear on radiographs.

Routine radiographs still may not be enough to diagnose subtalar joint instability. Broden described a technique to assess the congruity of the anterior, medial, and posterior facets, which is possible by positioning the leg in such a way that applies stress to an inverted rearfoot. In obtaining this view the foot is internally rotated approximately 40°, the beam is pointed at the center of the talonavicular joint, and the tube is angled 20° to 50°. Brantigan and colleagues[18] used Broden's stress view on 3 patients to diagnose subtalar joint instability; the study included 1 control. All 3 patients complained of symptoms of lateral instability. Though the study size was too small to provide significance, Brantigan and colleagues were able to show that when compared with the control, the symptomatic patients had an average of 19° more subtalar joint inversion.

Controversy about the Broden stress view does exist. Louwerens and colleagues[19] obtained inversion-stress Broden radiographs in 33 patients while using the asymptomatic side as a control. These investigators also studied 10 control patients who were completely asymptomatic. The study was unable to correlate increased amounts of subtalar joint motion with pain/instability; they found a wide range of subtalar joint motion in symptomatic as well as asymptomatic patients.[19]

Often it is necessary to obtain other modalities to evaluate the subtalar joint and surrounding structures, and MRI is especially helpful when the physical examination and radiographic studies do not match up. MRI allows for evaluation of periarticular cartilaginous and ligamentous structures that may be contributing to joint pain. It is a good modality to assess bone marrow edema as well as cartilage loss. If there is a suspicion of avascular necrosis MRI should be obtained to evaluate the extent, especially when fusion is being considered, as it has been shown that the extent of avascular necrosis correlates directly with the rate of nonunion.[2–5,20–23]

CT is yet another option that allows one to assess the subtalar joint. A CT scan allows one to better evaluate the quality of bone as well as look at osseous pathology of the joint that may not necessarily be visualized on a radiograph.

SURGICAL MANAGEMENT

Intravenous sedation or general anesthesia is used in conjunction with a regional popliteal or ankle block for this procedure. Patients receive a prophylactic antibiotic before the surgery. If used, a thigh tourniquet is placed after induction of anesthesia. The patient may be positioned supine with a hip bump or beanbag used to place the operative lower extremity in a lateral position. Choice of incision placement is based on the pathology. The commonly used lateral horizontal incision is placed for good visualization of the subtalar joint. The incision extends from the fibular malleolus distally to the calcaneocuboid joint lying just dorsal to the sural nerve and peroneal tendons. A lateral extensile incision may be preferred if the patient has had previous calcaneal fracture fixation.

Sharp and blunt dissection then proceeds through the subcutaneous tissue to the level of the deep fascia. If there are communicating nerve branches between the sural nerve and the intermediate dorsal cutaneous nerve across the field, they may be excised so as to avoid subsequent neuropraxia or neuritis associated with attempted retraction. The deep fascia and extensor retinaculum are then identified. The subtalar joint should then be manipulated to identify the sinus tarsi and the lateral process of the talus. Care should be taken to retract the sural nerve. The peroneal tendon sheath should be identified and protected. The L-shaped deep fascia incision is started vertically just anterior to the lateral process of the talus directed plantarly to the level of the calcaneus, then it curves distally around the inferior edge of the extensor digitorum muscle belly. The deep fascia, extensor digitorum muscle belly, and periosteum are then dissected free to expose the sinus tarsi and the posterior facet. The muscle belly may be tagged with suture to aid in retraction and final closure. The vertical aspect of the deep fascia incision is extended proximally as needed to properly visualize the posterior facet.

A bone rongeur or sharp dissection should then be used to evacuate the sinus tarsi and resect the interosseous ligament, thereby exposing the middle facet. The peroneal retinaculum is incised, and tendon sheath and the peroneal tendons are retracted plantarly and posteriorly away from the lateral malleolus. The calcaneofibular ligament and lateral talocalcaneal ligament are then incised and the surrounding soft tissue is released. Sayre elevators, osteotomes, and laminar spreaders are useful in gaining further access to the subtalar joint.

Cartilage is resected from talar and calcaneal articular surfaces. Without rearfoot deformity, minimal bone may be resected with the use of curettes, curved osteotomes, or flexible osteotomes. Minimal bone resection helps to retain the contours of the joint, which promotes better apposition of the talus and calcaneus; this is favorable for bone healing. Curved and flexible osteotomes help to resect the curved posterior facet. When resecting cartilage along the medial aspect of the posterior facet, care should be taken to avoid the medial neurovascular structures. Concluding cartilage resection with a curette is safer for the medial aspect of the posterior facet resection and for removal of the subchondral bone plate. An option used by many surgeons is subchondral drilling with a 0.062 Kirschner wire to promote bleeding at the arthrodesis site in lieu of a rotary burr.

If rearfoot position must be corrected, a bone wedge can be removed. The base of the resected wedge would be placed laterally for correction of rearfoot varus while a medially based wedge would resect to correct rearfoot valgus. Another option would be adding an autograft or allograft wedge to correct the hindfoot position. Resection versus graft application is based on surgeon's preference and whether wedge resection would lead to too much loss of height.

The joint is then positioned in a neutral position while cupping the heel or dorsiflexing the foot. The guide pin is placed and subtalar joint position is assessed under fluoroscopy. Fixation is often achieved with the use of a single percutaneous cannulated 6.5 mm screw directed from dorsal distal at the talar neck to plantar proximal across the posterior facet (**Fig. 2**). Alternatively, the screw can be inserted from proximal plantar to distal dorsal. Some surgeons may opt to apply a second screw or sometimes even a staple to counteract any rotational forces (**Figs. 3** and **4**).

Fusion of the subtalar joint may also be done arthroscopically. The use of a thigh tourniquet is recommended however, ankle distraction is not utilized. Lateral decubitus position is ideal for access via the anterolateral and posterolateral portals. A 2.7 mm scope is used to visualize the subtalar joint. A shaver is used to remove all synovitis and the use of burr, shavers and curettes are utilized in order to remove all the cartilage.

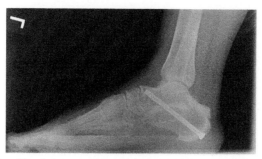

Fig. 2. Post operative film demonstrating STJ fusion utilizing a single screw.

Upon removal of the cartilage, 1-2 mm of subchondral bone is resected to expose cancellous bone. The talar and calcaneal surfaces are then fenestrated. Screw fixation is then inserted as stated above.

After a final fluoroscopic assessment, a layered closure is performed. A drain should be placed, if deemed necessary, after deflating the tourniquet.

COMPLICATIONS

Edema, hematoma, seroma, dehiscence, ulceration, and nerve damage can occur. Proper dissection and closure technique can minimize these complications.

Of course, patient compliance is a crucial component in the healing process. Soft-tissue infection should be immediately addressed with antibiotics, wound care, and surgical debridement if necessary to avoid progression to osteomyelitis. Patients must remain non–weight bearing as instructed. Patients would ideally also refrain from smoking during the crucial postoperative period.

As with any arthrodesis, nonunion, delayed union, and malunion are possible. Good surgical technique and rigid fixation will help to achieve the desired outcome. A hyper-trophic nonunion may require the use of an external bone stimulator whereas an atro-phic nonunion may require a second trip to the operating room. This visit would require resection of inactive bone or pseudoarthrosis, and application of demineralized bone matrix, allograft, or autograft. Additional internal fixation may be required as well. A malunion would require a revision of the fusion, osteotomies of adjacent bones, or the use accommodative orthotics for minor deformities.

Bone graft usage may lead to failure or fracture of the graft, nonunion, and residual valgus deformity. It is possible that the graft may not be incorporated, which would require a revisional procedure. Residual valgus deformity can possibly be treated by

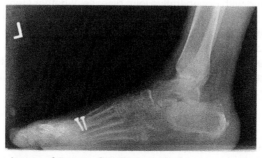

Fig. 3. Pre operative image of 2 screw fixation.

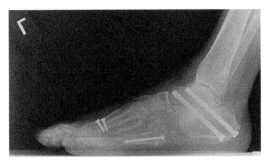

Fig. 4. Post operative image of 2 screw fixation.

bracing or orthotics, depending on the patient's degree of discomfort and readiness for further surgical intervention.

Painful retained hardware may lead to the need for eventual hardware removal. The newly fused subtalar joint will lead to decreased motion in the adjacent joints, as previously discussed, and this may in turn lead to arthritis of these neighboring joints.

POSTOPERATIVE MANAGEMENT

After a subtalar arthrodesis procedure, patients are often observed overnight for pain control. Immediately following the procedure, the patient is placed in a posterior splint. After some time the pain is controlled and the patient can be discharged from the hospital, and a below-knee cast is applied to the affected lower extremity. At this time, patients are instructed to be non–weight bearing. At about 3 weeks postoperatively, sutures can be removed if the wound site has healed, and patients can bear partial weight to the heel of the below-knee cast. At approximately 6 weeks postoperatively, patients can transition to a soft cast and CAM boot. At about 10 weeks, patients came begin to transition into normal shoe gear.[2] Throughout the postoperative course, routine radiographs should be taken in the lateral and Broden subtalar views to visualize the healing progression. If the patient complains of stiffness and weakness in the affected extremity after the 10 weeks postoperative period, physical therapy can be recommended for 3 to 4 weeks.

DISCUSSION

Isolated subtalar joint arthrodesis is an acceptable procedure for subtalar joint pathology, which specifically involves pain and rearfoot deformity localized to the subtalar joint, exclusive of all others. Painful debilitating frontal and transverse plane motion is associated with degenerative joint disease, whether stemming from trauma, congenital deformity, or long-standing tendon dysfunction. It has been shown that isolated fusions do affect adjacent joints, but not to a debilitating degree. Patients benefit from the improved quality of life with a greater ability to complete activities of daily living. On comprehensive consideration the authors have come to the conclusion that isolated subtalar joint fusion is a feasible surgical option when no other adjacent joints are affected.

REFERENCES

1. Astion D, Deland J, Otis J, et al. Motion of the hindfoot after simulated arthrodesis. J Bone Joint Surg Am 1997;79:241–6.

2. Easley ME, Hans-Jorg T, Schon LC, et al. Isolated subtalar arthrodesis. J Bone Joint Surg Am 2000;82(5):613–24.
3. Isherwood I. A radiological approach to the subtalar joint. J Bone Joint Surg Br 1961;43:566–74.
4. Muraro GM, Carvajal PF. Arthroscopic arthrodesis of subtalar joint. Foot Ankle Clin N Am 2011;16:83–90.
5. Diprimio R, Hirsch BE. Lower extremity anatomy manual. 2008. p. 110–5.
6. Donatelli RA. The biomechanics of the foot and ankle. FA Davis Co; 1996.
7. Kapandji IA. The physiology of the joints, vol.2. The lower limb. Churchill Livingstone, Longman group 2nd edition. 1970.
8. Wright DG, Desai SM, Henderson WH. Action of the subtalar and ankle joint complex during the stance phase of walking. J Bone Joint Surg Am 1964;46: 361–82.
9. Williams PL, Warwick R. Gray's anatomy. Edinburgh (United Kingdom): Churchill Livingstone; 1980.
10. Hicks JH. The mechanics of the foot. 1: the joints. J Anat 1953;87:345–57.
11. Leardini A, Stagni R, O'Connor JJ. Mobility of the subtalar joint in the intact ankle complex. J Biomech 2001;34(6):805–9.
12. Leardini A, O'Connor JJ, Catani F, et al. Kinematics of the human ankle complex in passive flexion; a single degree of freedom system. J Biomech 1999;32(2): 111–8.
13. Shephard E. Tarsal movements. J Bone Joint Surg Br 1951;33(2):258–63.
14. Keefe DT, Haddad SL. Subtalar instability: etiology, diagnosis and management. Foot Ankle Clin N Am 2002;7:577–609.
15. Therman H, Zwipp H, Tscherne H. Treatment algorithm for chronic ankle and subtalar instability. Foot Ankle Int 1997;18:163–9.
16. Gamble FO, Yale I. Clinical foot roentgenology: an illustrated hand book. Baltimore (MD): Williams & Wilkins; 1966.
17. LaPorta GA, Scarlet J. Radiographic changes in the pronated and supinated foot, a statistical analysis. J Am Podiatry Assoc 1977;76(5):334–8.
18. Brantigan JW, Pedegana LR, Lippert FG. Instability of the subtalar joint: diagnosis by stress tomography in three cases. J Bone Joint Surg Am 1977;59:321–4.
19. Louwerens JW, Ginai AZ, van Linge B, et al. Stress radiography of the talocrural and subtalar joints. Foot Ankle Int 1995;16:148–55.
20. Albert, A, Deleu PA, Leemrijse T, et al. Posterior arthroscopic subtalar arthrodesis: Ten cases at one-year follow up. Cliniques Universitaires Saint-Luc, Saint-Luc Academic Hospitals Avenue Hippocrate. 2011;10:1200.
21. Huang PJ, Fu YC, Cheng YM, et al. Subtalar arthrodesis for late sequelae of calcaneal fractures: fusion in situ versus fusion with sliding corrective osteotomy. Foot Ankle Int 1999;20(3):166–70.
22. Sammargo GJ, Tablante EB. Subtalar arthrodesis. Clin Orthop Relat Res 1998; 349(4):73–80.
23. Thermann H, Hufner T, Schratt E, et al. Long term results of subtalar fusions after operative versus non-operative treatment of os calcis fractures. Foot Ankle 1999; 20(7):408–15.

Calcaneocuboid Arthrodesis

Mohsen Barmada, DPM[a], Howard S. Shapiro, DPM[b],*,
Steven F. Boc, DPM[b,c]

KEYWORDS

• Calcaneocuboid joint • Arthrodesis • Lateral column

The calcaneocuboid joint is stable, even although multiple conditions might affect the joint, ranging from osteoarthritis to fracture, subluxation, and dislocation. Calcaneocuboid arthrodesis is more commonly performed as an adjunct procedure with other rearfoot procedures such as triple arthrodesis and is less used as isolated fusion. This article reviews the main conditions of the lateral column and calcaneocuboid joint in particular. The surgical technique for isolated calcaneocuboid arthrodesis is discussed.[1–4]

ANATOMY OF THE CALCANEOCUBOID JOINT

The calcaneocuboid joint is formed by the posterior surface of the cuboid and the anterior surface of the calcaneous. Along with the talocalcaneonavicular joint, it forms a complex known as the transverse tarsal joint.

Classification

The calcaneocuboid joint (also known as one-half of the Chopart joint) is a synovial, saddle, or sellar joint. Its articular areas are the posterior surface of the cuboid and the anterior surface of the calcaneus.

Ligaments

Capsular
The dorsal calcaneocuboid ligament runs from the lateral surface of the calcaneus to the dorsal surface of the cuboid. This is a weak ligament.

The plantar calcaneocuboid ligament extends from the anterior tubercle of the calcaneus to the cuboid, plantar surface, posterior to promontory. This ligament is short and wide and thickens the capsule.

[a] Hahnemann University Hospital, 235 North Broad Street, Suite 300, Philadelphia, PA 19107, USA
[b] Podiatric Medicine and Surgery Residency Program, Hahnemann University Hospital, 235 North Broad Street, Suite 300, Philadelphia, PA 19107, USA
[c] Department of Surgery, Drexel University College of Medicine, Philadelphia, PA, USA
* Corresponding author.
E-mail address: poddytrained@gmail.com

Clin Podiatr Med Surg 29 (2012) 77–89
doi:10.1016/j.cpm.2011.11.002
0891-8422/12/$ – see front matter © 2012 Elsevier Inc. All rights reserved.

podiatric.theclinics.com

Extracapsular

The long plantar ligament is the longest ligament in the foot and one of the longest in the body. It is separated from the plantar calcaneocuboid ligament by fatty tissue. Posteriorly, it is attached to the plantar surface of the calcaneus between the tuberosity and the anterior tubercle. Distally, it is attached to the promontory of the cuboid. Superficial fibers pass forward, forming the roof over the peroneal sulcus called the peroneal sheath. Superficial fibers continue, attaching to the bases of the second, third, fourth, and sometimes fifth metatarsals.

Bifurcate ligament

The calcaneocuboid part of the bifurcate ligament is attached to the lateral end of the sulcus calcanei, passing distal to the medial surface of the cuboid.

Blood Supply

The blood supply is through the branches of the lateral tarsal and lateral plantar arteries.

Innervations

The lateral terminal branch of the deep peroneal nerve supplies the calcaneocuboid joint. The superficial peroneal and lateral plantar nerves occasionally supply the joint as well.

BIOMECHANICS OF THE CALCANEOCUBOID JOINT

The midtarsal joint oblique axis is the main axis that runs through the calcaneocuboid articulation of the midtarsal joint. The midtarsal joint oblique axis passes medial, anterior, and dorsal, through the center of the head of the talus and out through the lower, lateral, and middle portion of the calcaneus.

The midtarsal joint oblique axis lies 52° from the sagittal plane and 57° from the transverse plane. The amount of motion in the frontal plane is minuscule. The amount of freedom in the sagittal and transverse planes allows for the oblique axis to move the foot in dorsiflexion/plantarflexion and abduction/adduction, respectively. This movement allows the forefoot to properly compensate for problems in the ankle joint, which is sagittal plane dominant.

GENERAL INDICATIONS FOR JOINT FUSION

General indications for joint fusions are multiple. However, the main components are related to injuries, diseases, or congenital defects. First, injuries could be simple or compound fractures and may be associated with dislocation. Second, diseases may affect the function of the joint in 2 ways. The first way is directly by damaging the articular surfaces, which results in a decrease of the fibrous tissue. An example of this is osteoarthritis. The second way is indirectly. For example, disease such as anterior poliomyelitis or upper motor neuron disorder may be associated with instability of the joint. The third way includes congenital defects such as congenital absence of 1 or more of the foot bones.[5,6]

Indications for calcaneocuboid arthrodesis[1,2,7–14]

1. Correction of deformity (congenital such as arthrogryposis or acquired)
2. Degenerative joint disease
3. Flexible or rigid acquired flat foot
4. Neglected/relapsed club foot

5. Cerebral palsy
6. Posttraumatic reconstruction.

Factors that play an important role resulting in arthrodesis include

1. Total removal of the articular cartilage
2. Careful attention to maintain the contour of the surfaces. Careful attention should also be paid to the structures surrounding the joint to ensure that their proper function and relationship are intact after fusion.[7,15]

As mentioned earlier, one of the main indications for calcaneocuboid fusion is correction of flat foot deformity. Logel and colleagues[2] described lengthening of lateral column by calcaneocuboid distraction arthrodesis and tendon transfer on 10 fresh frozen cadaver lower extremity specimens. Because lengthening of the lateral column increases the pressure on the lateral column, creating forefoot varus, these investigators added first metatarsocuneiform arthrodesis, reducing the pressure on the lateral column and elevating the medial arch of the foot and all the radiographic parameters, with noticeable improvement.

Another prospective study by van der Krans and colleagues[8] applied calcaneocuboid distraction arthrodesis, posterior tibial tendon augmentation, and percutaneous Achilles tendon lengthening to 20 patients (20 feet) with adult acquired flexible flatfoot. The mean age was 55 (30–66) years and the group comprised 16 women and 4 men. Arthrodesis of the first cuneiform-metatarsal joint was performed in 8 patients and naviculocuneiform arthrodesis was performed in 2 patients to correct the forefoot supination and hallux valgus. The foot function index and American Orthopedic Foot and Ankle Society (AOFAS) Clinical Rating Index hindfoot score were obtained preoperatively and postoperatively. Patients were followed over 25 months. The results were complete pain relief and increase in daily activity in 17 patients. The satisfaction rate ranged from good to excellent in 15 patients. Pain at the distraction site was noted in 3 patients only. Significant improvement was observed on radiographic parameters in dorsoplantar and lateral talometatarsal angle in addition to ground-navicular distance. The technique was performed with 0.8-cm to 1.0-cm distractions and an iliac crest graft was used. Fixation was achieved with a cervical H-plate from Synthes (Synthes Inc., West Chester, PA, USA) with 2 distal and 2 proximal cortical screws. Postoperatively, all patients were immobilized with a non–weight-bearing cast for 4 weeks followed by a weight-bearing cast for another 4 weeks. Next, a cam walker was used for the last 4 weeks. Orthotics were prescribed at 5 months. On radiographic studies, union was noticed in 16 feet within 3 months and in 1 foot within 4 months and 1 foot in 5 months. Nonunion was noticed in 2 feet only. Three patients complained of paresthesia or anesthesia in the sural nerve area.

Another study by Kitaoka[3] viewed the role of calcaneocuboid distraction arthrodesis in posterior tibial tendon dysfunction and flatfoot. In the early stages, a soft tissue procedure was used. For example, flexor digitorum longus tendon transfer might benefit the patient. In late stages of the disorder associated with rigid deformity and hindfoot arthritis, arthrodesis plays a main role.

The last scenario is when a patient is in the late stages but stiffness is not associated; those patients benefit from calcaneocuboid distraction arthrodesis. Anderson and Davis[3] reported the results of calcaneocuboid distraction arthrodesis in patients with acquired flat foot associated with posterior tibial dysfunction. One of 13 patients developed nonunion, and most patients reported improvement in foot alignment and symptoms.

Calcaneocuboid distraction arthrodesis may be associated with limitations and complications. The main limitation is that calcaneocuboid distraction arthrodesis includes using a bone graft, which might be large enough to prolong the healing process.[2]

Three main complications are associated with calcaneocuboid distraction arthrodesis: nonunion, malunion, and stress fracture of the lateral column.[1,3,8,16] In a study performed by Thomas and colleagues, 17 feet were used. Two nonunion, 3 delayed unions, 3 graft stress fractures, and 1 fifth metatarsal stress fracture were reported.[3] Another study by Chi and colleagues of 12 feet with isolated calcaneocuboid distraction arthrodesis reported 2 nonunions.[3] However, these investigators also reported study arthrodesis, resulting in 8 nonunions.[3]

Posttraumatic calcaneocuboid fusion is a broad subject. Many studies have been performed on calcaneal trauma and the percentage of calcaneocuboid joint involvement. Studies have shown that the calcaneocuboid joint is involved in 33% to 76% of calcaneal fractures. In a study of 553 calcaneal fractures prepared by Zwipp and colleagues, 59.7% were associated with calcaneocuboid joint involvement.[5] Clinically, patients with calcaneocuboid joint involvement have the same level of pain as patients without calcaneocuboid joint involvement according to Ebraheim and colleagues.[5] However, walking on a rough surface causes a problem. Also subtalar joint involvement is difficult to rule out clinically. Generally, severe trauma is mostly associated with calcaneocuboid joint involvement.

Other conditions that might affect the calcaneocuboid joint and result in fusion include[1,3,8]:

1. Forefoot or midfoot adductus, which applies more mechanical pressure to lateral columns.
2. Pronation deformity, which might be associated with hypermobile calcaneocuboid joint or unstable midtarsal joint.
3. Cuboid syndrome or subluxation of the calcaneocuboid joint, which might be caused by many factors such as firing of the peroneal tendon in external or internal rotation and results in more stress applied to the calcaneocuboid joint and subluxation at the end. On the other hand, cuboid syndrome is an inflammation of the calcaneocuboid joint caused by mild malposition of that joint. Isolated subluxation or dislocation of the calcaneocuboid joint without fracture is not common.
4. Direct injury to the ligaments of calcaneocuboid joint might occur and is usually associated with supination mechanism.
5. Biomechanical disorder or idiopathic lateral column pain, when no cause can be found to explain the calcaneocuboid joint pain. In this case, gait analysis with complete biomechanical examination of the foot is important. Furthermore, orthotics might be considered as a milestone for treatment.
6. Lateral band release of the plantar fascia caused by severe dissection during plantar fasciotomy procedure usually results in applying more pressure to the calcaneocuboid joint and manifests as lateral column pain.

NONINVASIVE TREATMENT OF CALCANEOCUBOID JOINT DISORDER

Before considering surgical intervention for lateral column and calcaneocuboid joint disease, conservative modalities of treatment are highly recommended. These modalities include padding of the cuboid to offload the pressure on the calcaneocuboid joint.[1] In addition, custom-molded orthotics plays an important role similar to cuboid padding. Repositioning the calcaneocuboid joint in normal alignment, the maneuver to realign the joint is called black snake heel whip.[1] This maneuver is performed by having the patient standing flexing the knee in the affected limb to 90°. The physician stands behind the patient and holds the forefoot of the patient with their fingers and positions their thumbs over each other on the medial plantar aspect of the cuboid bone. Next, the physician manipulates the foot like a whip in a fast movement to reposition the cuboid laterally and dorsally. A pop noise indicates that the calcaneocuboid joint has been repositioned. Low-dye strapping is then used to keep the alignment intact.

Prolotherapy[1] is one of the methods to treat chronic calcaneocuboid subluxation by strengthening the capsule and ligaments of the joint. It is an injection of dextrose, anesthetic, and phenol. The mechanism is to inject through the joint capsule, which results in sclerosis and increases the blood supply. A pseudoarthrosis develops and subluxation improves.

Calcaneocuboid Arthrodesis

Fusion of the calcaneocuboid joint can be considered after all noninvasive methods of treatment have failed. Usually, triple arthrodesis is indicated when a patient has midtarsal or subtalar joint pain associated with calcaneocuboid joint arthrosis.[1]

Although isolated calcaneocuboid joint arthrodesis is believed to end with degenerative arthritic changes in the surrounding joints, much success has been reported by performing isolated calcaneocuboid joint fusion. Thomas and colleagues performed 5 isolated fourth and fifth metatarsal base cuboid fusions and 15 isolated calcaneocuboid fusions.[1] As a result, some patients who had distal fusion developed pain at the calcaneocuboid joint. However, patients who had calcaneocuboid joint fusion did not report any pain. The distal joints adjust and function better, considering that the main motion in the lateral column comes from the fourth and fifth metatarsal cuboid joint more than the calcaneocuboid joint. Also Achilles lengthening should be considered when performing lateral column fusion to avoid posterior equines. It is helpful to use an injection in the distal or proximal joints to locate the source of the pain in the lateral column.[1,8]

Abduction of the foot might develop after calcaneocuboid fusion, but usually patients function normally without the talonavicular joint being affected.[1]

Surgical technique

The patient is placed on the operating table in a supine position. A blanket is placed under the ipsilateral hip for support.[7,8,15,17] A pneumatic thigh tourniquet is applied for hemostasis and inflated to 350 mm Hg for the duration of the case. Next, the foot and ankle are scrubbed, draped, and prepared in the usual aseptic manner. A longitudinal linear skin incision is made along the lateral aspect of the foot over the calcaneocuboid joint starting from the tip of the fibula and extending to the base of the fourth metatarsal. Care is taken to retract the sural nerve with any branches. Then, the deep fascia is dissected to expose the extensor digitorum brevis and peroneal tendon sheath. The extensor digitorum brevis is dissected from its origin after opening the capsule and the muscle is retracted distal to the calcaneocuboid joint. Then the peroneal tendon sheath is split longitudinally and reflected plantarly.

Usually, a freer elevator is used to maintain retraction of all soft tissue structures and to be inserted within the calcaneocuboid joint. The location of the joint is confirmed using fluoroscopy. After the calcaneocuboid joint is exposed, a sagittal saw or sharp osteotome or curette is used to remove the articular cartilage from the proximal surface of the cuboid and the distal surface of the calcaneus. Care should be taken to maintain the saddle shape of the cuboid-calcaneal joint. If a sagittal saw is used, the blade should be placed parallel to the transverse and sagittal planes. After removing a 1-mm to 1.5-mm layer of subchondral bone, the arthrodesis site is exposed with proper bone-to-bone apposition and cancellous bone surfaces. A key elevator can be used to reflect the periosteum and to expose the calcaneocuboid joint. It is important to confirm that the joint capsule is dissected completely to have better exposure of the joint.

Before starting the internal fixation, a small drill of 1.6-mm wire is used to fenestrate bone surfaces both at the cuboid and at the calcaneus. A laminar spreader can be inserted in the joint to get better exposure for fenestration and deep drilling to increase vascularity during the healing process.

Several methods can be followed to perform internal fixation of the calcaneocuboid joint. Using 4.0-mm cannulated screws is 1 method that can be used for fixation. Usually, 1 screw is inserted proximally to distally from the anterior process of the calcaneus, extending in an oblique direction to the cuboid, and the other screw is inserted in the opposite direction distally to proximally and crossing the first screw.

The second method of fixation is power staples. This method is usually applied to soft bone and patients with rheumatoid arthritis. Attention should be directed to the arrangement of staples around the joint to obtain the proper stabilization.

The third method of fixation is plate fixation. More stability to the fusion site can be applied by using plate fixation. Usually, an H-plate with locking screws is used to provide interfragmentary compression. The plate is placed dorsolaterally overlying the calcaneocuboid joint and the 3.5-mm distal lateral screws are inserted using the proper technique followed by the 3.5-mm distal medial screw. Care should be taken to ensure that the screws remained within the cuboid under fluoroscopy. The 2 3.5-mm proximal screws are then inserted within the plate. Care should be taken to ensure that the calcaneal screws do not enter the subtalar joint under fluoroscopy. The surgical site is then flushed with copious amounts of sterile saline and a bone graft is inserted to fill the minimal void within the calcaneocuboid joint. The arthrodesis site should be inspected before closing the wound. The extensor digitorum brevis and peroneal tendon sheath can be repaired to the underlying periosteum by using absorbable suture. Also an absorbable suture, such as 2.0 and 3.0 vicryl, can be used for capsule and subcutaneous closure. Skin can be closed with nonabsorbable suture such as 4.0 prolene. During closure, care should be taken not to disturb the sural nerve, particularly when suturing the subcutaneous layers. Injection of 0.5% bupivacaine postoperatively is recommended to maintain postoperative pain relief. A sterile dressing is applied to the incision site. Afterward, compression dressing with a below-knee posterior fiberglass splint is placed.

Postoperative management

A popliteal block can be applied in the recovery room to provide postoperative analgesia.[7,8,15] Instructions are given to the patient to be non–weight bearing and to ice and elevate the operative limb. Prescriptions for pain control medications are indicated. Two weeks postoperatively, the sutures can be removed and a below-knee cast applied. Nonweight bearing continues for 6 weeks from the date of surgery. A cast change and radiographs are indicated at 6 weeks postoperatively. If radiographs show progressive union, the patient can start weight bearing with the cast. Twelve weeks postoperatively, radiographs are obtained again. If proper union has occurred, the patient can start weight bearing as tolerated with a removable walker boot. When the patient is pain-free or fully weight bearing, physical therapy is indicated.

Complications

The most common complication after calcaneocuboid arthrodesis is delayed union or nonunion. Many factors may play a role including smoking, early weight bearing, noncompliance, equinus contracture, or improper fixation. Other possible complications include entrapment of the sural nerve and its branches, stress fracture, peroneal tendonitis, hardware failure, and arthritic changes in the surrounding joints.[3,7,8,15,18]

CASE REPORT

A 55-year-old woman presented for evaluation, care, and treatment of the left ankle and left foot. She remembered banging the lateral aspect of her left foot. She pointed around the region of the fibula, peroneal muscles, and sinus tarsi area. The area was sore to touch, palpation, and with shoe gear. There was a significant amount of swelling, with venous insufficiency and stasis changes noted to the skin. There was a significant amount of edema, erythema, and rubor. There were no signs of cellulitis or infection. No open lesions were noted. The patient had a significant amount of muscle guarding, stiffness, and tenderness. The vascular examination was intact. The dorsalis pedis and posterior tibial pulses were 2/4. Cap refills were 3 seconds. The neurologic examination revealed hypersensitivity along the sural nerve. The right ankle was asymptomatic. The radiographic evaluation showed no acute signs of fracture/dislocation, although there were some cortical changes around the fibula, distal aspect, and around the malleolar region. This finding is consistent with a bone contusion/stress reaction. Additional findings included decreased joint space in the ankle, some osteoarthritic changes, bone spurring across the dorsum of the foot, slight pes planus foot type, and no occult signs of fracture/dislocation or infectious processes otherwise indicated. The review of systems was clear. The medical history was unremarkable. There were no known allergies. The patient stated that she had broken bones in her ankle. The patient never smoked or drank and had no history of illicit drug use. Her family history included diabetes, stroke, and cancer. The cardiovascular examination was normal. The respiratory examination was also normal. The gastrointestinal and genitourinary examination were both normal. The muscular skeletal examination was within normal limits.

The assessment was

1. Bone contusion injury
2. Possible ankle sprain/strain
3. Peroneal tendonitis
4. Bursitis of the ankle
5. Venous/stasis with swelling.

The plan was

1. Radiographs taken of the left foot and ankle
2. Injection to the left ankle, performed with 1 mL of lidocaine plain, 1 mL of Marcaine plain, and 0.5 mL of dexamethasone phosphate
3. Cast immobilization performed
4. Prescription given for nonsteroidal antiinflammatory medication
5. Magnetic resonance imaging (MRI) ordered to evaluate the ankle and tendon/ligament
6. Return to clinic in 4 weeks for follow-up care and treatment.

In the following 4 weeks, the patient presented to the office with minimum relief from previous treatment. The MRI report showed left foot and ankle degenerative joint disease, calcaneocuboid degenerative joint disease with possible osteomyelitis, and a soft tissue mass at the calcaneocuboid joint.

The patient underwent surgery for left ankle arthroscopy, a bone biopsy of the left calcaneus and cuboid, application of external fixation (minirail with 2 pins extending into the posterior calcaneus, one-tenth extending into the cuboid), and excision of the soft tissue mass at the calcaneocuboid joint. The pathology result showed chronic osteomyelitis in both calcaneal and cuboid biopsies. The soft tissue mass showed fibrosis with chronic inflammation. Microbiology was negative (**Figs. 1–3**).

The patient presented for evaluation, care, and treatment 10 days after calcaneocuboid resection with a history of possible osteomyelitis. The patient was stable. Neurovascular status was intact. The skin edges were coapted. Some pain and swelling were noted. Radiographs were taken of the left foot. Clinically, patient had no signs of infection or drainage externally. A sterile dressing and posterior splint were applied, and offloading the left foot with rest, ice, compression, and elevation was continued. The patient was to return for follow-up in 1 month.

The patient presented 1 month later for evaluation, care, and treatment. She had left calcaneocuboid distraction secondary to a history of osteomyelitis, which was stable. Neurovascular status was intact. The skin edges were coapted. There were no signs of infection. A posterior splint had been used to stabilize the foot, ankle, and leg and while weight bearing or walking. We are not sure where the infectious processes came from, but it was all stable. There were no signs of progression, and it was probably just a chronic type of infection. At this point, we planned to continue stabilizing the ankle and foot and sending her for possible surgical repair and removal of hardware with possible fusion and use of internal/external fixations. There was no progression of osteomyelitis. We continued local wound care only. The patient was to stay off the extremity and to continue antiinflammatory and pain medications as needed. Radiographs of the left foot (3 views) showed good alignment, good positioning, and good healing. The patient was to return in 2 weeks for follow-up.

On next follow-up, the patient presented with stable postoperative status, stable wound sites, intact frame, and no signs of infection or drainage. Radiographs of the left foot (3 views) showed good healing. The patient was given instructions to continue non–weight bearing and scheduled for surgery in 2 weeks for removal of external fixation and calcaneocuboid joint arthrodesis with bone graft application. The patient underwent surgery. The external fixation frame was removed and the calcaneocuboid joint was fused by using a plate with 4 locking screws and a bone graft application. The patient tolerated the procedure well; she was instructed to remain non–weight bearing, and prescriptions for postoperative pain management were given (**Figs. 4–6**).

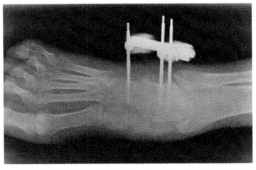

Fig. 1. Patient status after left foot application of external fixation to the calcaneocuboid joint (anteroposterior view).

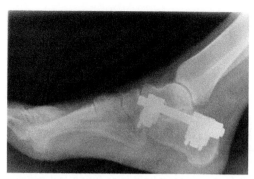

Fig. 2. Patient status after left foot application of external fixation to the calcaneocuboid joint (lateral view).

On the following postoperative visits, the patient was stable, neurovascular status was intact, skin edges were coapted, and there was no sign of infection. The patient reported some pain at the lateral aspect of the left foot, but only if she increased activity or weight bearing. Radiographs were taken and showed good alignment, good positioning, and good healing. Good stability was noted with no signs of fractural dislocation or infection.

Three weeks postoperatively, the sutures were removed and a short leg fiberglass cast was applied; the patient was advised to continue with pain medications as needed. Pain management was also discussed.

At the 5-week follow-up visit, the patient was noted to have restrictive and antalgic gait. Radiography showed delayed union, and a bone stimulator was recommended , with full instructions given to the patient regarding its use.

At 12 weeks postoperatively, it was noted that the patient had edema to the left foot and some stiffness when walking barefoot. The patient was able to balance in shoes. The incision at the lateral aspect was healed. Radiography showed a stable and aligned calcaneocuboid joint and intact hardware with no sign of fracture or infection. At this point, the patient was instructed to start gentle physical therapy exercises.

At the 16-week follow-up visit, the patient was improving on physical therapy, but she still had some pain and restriction in range of motion. Radiography showed incomplete fusion of the calcaneocuboid joint. The patient was able to walk, with some

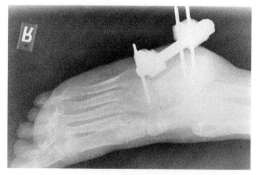

Fig. 3. Patient status after left foot application of external fixation to the calcaneocuboid joint (medial-oblique view).

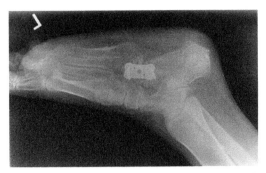

Fig. 4. Status after left foot calcaneocuboid joint fusion and removal of external fixation (medial-oblique view).

stiffness and edema if she was on her feet for an extended period of time. At this point, the patient was instructed to continue physical therapy with range-of-motion exercise and stretching, and to continue with limited activities as tolerated.

In the following weeks, the patient started to develop pain at the Lisfranc joint. She was sent for a computed tomography scan of the soft tissue window of the left foot, which showed demineralization and a questionable Lisfranc joint injury (separation of the Lisfranc area). There were fundamental changes within the first and second metatarsal cuneiforms consistent with Lisfranc injury and bone contusion. It was clear that the patient had first presented with an undiagnosed condition and disease, which we found by proper diagnostic testing. The patient had to be treated first by resection of the area and external fixation followed by closure of the area and use of internal fixation. The result has been some progressive changes in the midtarsal area and the tarsal regions, which are associated with tarsal-metatarsal dislocation. These are the signs and symptoms that are consistent with a Lisfranc injury. At this point, surgical intervention including open reduction with internal fixation to repair the medial and lateral column was discussed with the patient.

A month later, the patient presented with continuous pain and discomfort at the Lisfranc area and agreed to have surgical intervention. Two weeks after her previous visit, the patient had left foot Lisfranc joint fusion with medial column fusion and bone graft application. Fusion was performed by using a 3.5-mm screw (**Figs. 7–9**).

At the 1-week postoperative visit, the patient presented with pain and discomfort to the left foot. The cast was removed. The foot had moderate erythema and edema at

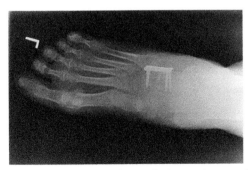

Fig. 5. Status after left foot calcaneocuboid joint fusion and removal of external fixation (anteroposterior view).

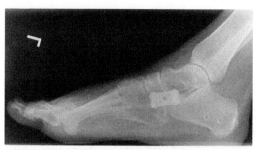

Fig. 6. Status after left foot calcaneocuboid joint fusion and removal of external fixation (lateral view).

the surgical site. There was some ecchymosis at the toes. The incision sites seemed to be healing well. No drainage, purulence, or any sign of infection was noted at the incision sites. However, there was an area of cellulitis on the dorsum of the foot. Radiographs of the left foot (3 views) showed that all hardware was in a good position and unchanged from the surgical date. Moderate soft tissue edema was noted. The patient was redressed with a dry, sterile dressing and placed back into a below-knee cast. She was instructed to keep non–weight bearing. She was also prescribed antibacterial medication for her cellulitis for 2 weeks, and pain medication.

In the following visit, the patient stated that the pain and discomfort had decreased. The cast was removed, and it was noted that the erythema and edema had significantly decreased. There was only a small area of erythema localized to the incision sites. No active drainage, purulence, or any sign of infection was noted. Edema was greatly decreased, as well as some of the ecchymosis on the digits. The patient was redressed with a dry, sterile dressing and placed back into a below-knee fiberglass cast. She was also instructed to keep non–weight bearing and to finish her antibacterial medication and to take pain medication as needed.

At 3 weeks postoperatively, the patient stated that she was still having mild pain and discomfort to the left foot. It was noted that she presented in a wheelchair with her cast clean, dry, and intact. On examination, the previous erythema had completely diminished. No drainage, purulence, or any sign of infection was noted. Both incision sites seemed to be well healed. No edema was noted. Radiographs of the left foot (3 views) showed that all hardware was in a good position and unchanged from previous radiographs. Incomplete union of the talonavicular joint was noted. The first

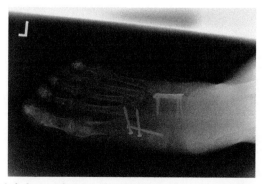

Fig. 7. Status after left foot Lisfranc and medial column fusion (anteroposterior view).

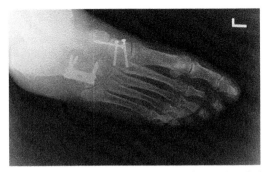

Fig. 8. Status after left foot Lisfranc and medial column fusion (medial-oblique view).

metatarsal-cuneiform seemed to be well fused. All sutures were removed and incision sites were reinforced with sterile strips. The patient was placed back into a below-knee fiberglass cast, with instructions to continue non–weight bearing to the left foot, to continue ice and elevation, and to take pain medication as needed.

At 6 weeks postoperatively, the patient presented with minimal pain and discomfort to the left foot. All incisions were well healed. No edema and no signs of infection were noted. There was mild pain on palpation over the previously fused surgical areas. The patient progressed into a supportive Unna boot, with a cam boot for guarded ambulation. The patient was also instructed to continue with moderation of activity. In the following visits, the patient continued to have pain improvement and progressed to a cam boot only. The Unna boot was removed. The patient started to ambulate better and gradually progressed to a regular shoe.

Case Discussion

The patient first presented with an undiagnosed and untreated previous injury to the left calcaneocuboid joint. Diagnostic tests showed degenerative disease in the calcaneocuboid joint in addition to chronic osteomyelitis in both cuboid and calcaneus bones. The patient underwent external fixation with anthrotomy of the calcaneocuboid joint. With continuous pain, the patient underwent for calcaneocuboid joint fusion. A few months later, she developed arthritic changes with dislocation at the distal and medial surrounding joints, which required fusion of those joints. In general, fusing 1 column placed more stress on the medial column and the adjacent joints. Other factors like chronic osteomyelitis can affect the healing process of the bones and joints.

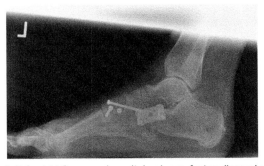

Fig. 9. Status after left foot Lisfranc and medial column fusion (lateral view).

SUMMARY

Calcaneocuboid arthrodesis can result from different causes. Care should be taken before fusing the joint by trying the other conservative methods and selecting the proper way of fixation, and also when choosing isolated calcaneocuboid arthrodesis versus double or triple arthrodesis.

REFERENCES

1. Chang TJ, Soomekh DJ. Lateral column fusions. Clin Podiatr Med Surg 2004; 21(1):129–39.
2. Logel KJ, Parks BG, Schon LC. Calcaneocuboid distraction arthrodesis and first metatarsocuneiform arthrodesis for correction of acquired flatfoot deformity in a cadaver model. Foot Ankle Int 2007;28(4):435–40.
3. Kitaoka HB, Kura H, Luo ZP, et al. Calcaneocuboid distraction arthrodesis for posterior tibial tendon dysfunction and flatfoot: a cadaveric study. Clin Orthop Relat Res 2000;(381):241–7.
4. Mcharo C, Ochsner P. Isolated bilateral recurrent dislocation of the calcaneocuboid joint. J Bone Joint Surg Br 1997;79(4):648–9.
5. Kinner B, Schieder S, Müller F, et al. Calcaneocuboid joint involvement in calcaneal fractures. J Trauma 2010;68(5):1192–9.
6. Glissan DJ. The indications for inducing fusion at the ankle joint by operation, with description of two successful techniques. Aust N Z J Surg 1949;19(1):64–71.
7. Mann RA. Arthrodesis of the foot and ankle. In: Coughlin MJ, Mann RA, Saltzman CL, et al, editors. Surgery of the foot and ankle. Philadelphia: Mosby Elsevier; 2007. p. 1087–123.
8. van der Krans A, Louwerens JW, Anderson P. Adult acquired flexible flatfoot, treated by calcaneocuboid distraction arthrodesis, posterior tibial tendon augmentation, and percutaneous Achilles tendon lengthening: a prospective outcome study of 20 patients. Acta Orthop 2006;77(1):156–63.
9. Jung HG, Myerson MS, Schon LC. Spectrum of operative treatments and clinical outcomes for atraumatic osteoarthritis of the tarsometatarsal joints. Foot Ankle Int 2007;28(4):482–9.
10. Adams E, Madden C. Cuboid subluxation: a case study and review of the literature. Curr Sports Med Rep 2009;8(6):300–7.
11. Adams SB Jr, Simpson AW, Pugh LI, et al. Calcaneocuboid joint subluxation after calcaneal lengthening for planovalgus foot deformity in children with cerebral palsy. J Pediatr Orthop 2009;29(2):170–4.
12. Kitaoka HB, Kura H, Luo ZP, et al. Calceocuboid distraction arthrodesis for posterior tibial tendon dysfunction and flatfoot. Clin Orthop 2000;381:241–7.
13. Anderson RB, Davis WH. Calcaneocuboid distraction arthrodesis for the treatment of the adult acquired flatfoot. Foot Ankle Clin 1996;1:279–94.
14. Blakeslee T, Morris J. Cuboid syndrome and the significance of midtarsal joint stability. J Am Podiatr Med Assoc 1987;77(12):638–42.
15. Grossman J. Calcaneal cuboid distraction arthrodesis. In: Chang TJ, editor. Master techniques in podiatric surgery: the foot and ankle. Philadelphia: Lippincott Williams & Wilkins; 2005. p. 323–31.
16. Flamme CH, Wulker N, Muller A, et al. Long-term follow-up after arthrodesis of the ankle and the hindfoot. Foot Ankle Surg 1997;3:21–8.
17. Deland JT, Otis JC, Lee KT, et al. Lateral column lengthening with calcaneocuboid fusion: Range of motion in the triple joint complex. Foot Ankle Int 1995;16:729–33.
18. Gallina J, Sands AK. Lateral-sided bony procedures. Foot Ankle Clin 2003;8(3):563–7.

Triple Arthrodesis

Albert M. D'Angelantonio, BSME, DPM[a,b,*],
Faith A. Schick, DPM[c,d], Neda Arjomandi, MS, DPM[e]

KEYWORDS

- Triple arthrodesis • Traumatic arthritis
- Degenerative joint disease • Tarsal coalitions

INDICATIONS

Edwin W. Ryerson first described triple arthrodesis in 1923 as a fusion of the talocalcaneal, talonavicular, and calcaneal cuboid joints.[1] The goal was to create a well-aligned, plantigrade, and stable foot for patients with deformity or progressive neurologic and arthritic conditions. This procedure should be reserved for instances when all conservative measures have been tried and failed, and a more limited surgical procedure will not afford appropriate pain relief and reduction of the deformity. In cases of a flexible deformity, consideration should first be given to those procedures that are joint sparing, such as tendon transfers or osteotomies.

The following is a list of indications for triple arthrodesis:

- Subtalar osteoarthritis with either talonavicular or calcaneocuboid degenerative joint disease
- Charcot-Marie-Tooth disease
- Polio residuals
- Peripheral nerve injuries with fixed deformities
- Cerebrovascular accident
- Painful flexible or fixed rheumatoid hindfoot deformities
- Symptomatic posttraumatic malalignment (ie, following a fracture of the talar neck with involvement of both the talar neck and subtalar joint), or with hindfoot joint instability
- Posttraumatic arthritis, most commonly seen following a fracture of the talus or calcaneus (**Fig. 1**)

[a] Kennedy University Hospital, Stratford, NJ 08084, USA
[b] Private Practice, Regional Foot and Ankle Specialists, 188 Fries Mill Road, Suite N-2, Turnersville, NJ 08012, USA
[c] Community Medical Center, Toms River, NJ 08755, USA
[d] Private Practice, 1163 Highway 37 West, Suite 2B, Toms River, NJ 08755, USA
[e] Kennedy Memorial Hospital, University Medical Center, Stratford, NJ 08084, USA
* Corresponding author. Private Practice, Regional Foot and Ankle Specialists, 188 Fries Mill Road, Suite N-2, Turnersville, NJ 08012.
E-mail address: aldangelo@comcast.net

Clin Podiatr Med Surg 29 (2012) 91–102
doi:10.1016/j.cpm.2011.09.004
0891-8422/12/$ – see front matter © 2012 Elsevier Inc. All rights reserved.

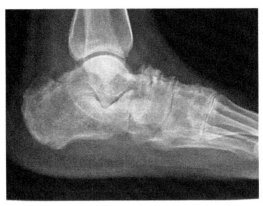

Fig. 1. Posttraumatic arthritis. Lateral view radiograph. Patient is status after calcaneocuboid fracture. Degenerative hindfoot arthritis is noted.

- Nonresectable calcaneonavicular or talocalcaneal coalition
- Posterior tibialis tendon dysfunction with a fixed deformity.[2–4]

CONTRAINDICATIONS

Contraindications for triple arthrodesis include any clinical situation that could be treated with a more limited fusion. It is important to isolate the affected joints. Initially this may be done through clinical examination and imaging evaluation. Alternatively, the affected joints may be isolated through the use of intra-articular lidocaine injections. Patients with peripheral vascular disease and blood supply inadequate for healing following surgery should not undergo the procedure. Preoperative evaluation by a vascular specialist is always advised when there is any question as to the patient's ability to heal. It is also not advisable to perform a triple arthrodesis on patients with neuroarthropathy or with systemic healing issues.

Advanced age and diabetes mellitus are not direct contraindications for triple arthrodesis, although it has implications for the postoperative care regimen.[3] Proper control of blood sugar is necessary to allow an optimal postoperative course.

PHYSIOLOGY AND PATHOMECHANICS

Evaluation of the foot in both standing and resting positions is imperative to patient evaluation. Usually, a varus hindfoot has a compensatory forefoot valgus with a plantarflexed first ray. In this case, additional procedures may be necessary to bring the foot in a plantigrade position following the triple arthrodesis. Claw toes may be present as well. Underlying neuromuscular disorders such as Charcot-Marie-Tooth disease or spinal lesions can cause a cavus foot type.

The hindfoot and forefoot are linked because they compensate for one another. A valgus hindfoot usually compensates with forefoot varus deformity and an abducted forefoot. This compensation is usually centralized around the Chopart joint. For this reason, there is little need for more distal surgery because much can be corrected simply with a triple arthrodesis. Sometimes in valgus foot the Achilles tendon becomes contracted. The Achilles tendon is shortened and calcaneus is laterally deviated. In such cases, the patient also has limited dorsiflexion of the ankle joint. If there is a rigid hindfoot deformity, it may not be possible to evaluate for contracture of the Achilles tendon before surgery. In instances such as this, evaluation of the need for either an Achilles tendon lengthening or gastrocnemius recession must be made during surgery.

Neutral foot weight bearing has 5° of hindfoot valgus. The flatfoot in the non–weight-bearing position has 5° of hindfoot valgus, but it compensates in weight bearing and has 17° of hindfoot valgus. The cavus foot in the non–weight-bearing position has 5° of hindfoot valgus, but in the weight-bearing position it compensates with 17° of hindfoot valgus.

The position of the foot with a respect to the entire lower extremity must be evaluated when preoperatively planning for triple arthrodesis.

The angle of the tibial mechanical axis and its relation to the forefoot should be considered. The tibial mechanical axis has 3 basic forms:

- Varus tibial mechanical axis
- Neutral tibial mechanical axis
- Valgus tibial mechanical axis

Preoperative valgus mechanical alignment and preoperative varus tibial alignment have an effect on the ultimate position of the foot after triple arthrodesis. Even if the tibial malalignment is not corrected, foot malalignment can be avoided, because the foot has been placed in a plantigrade position with respect to the preexisting proximal lower alignment. This concept comes into play when a patient is to undergo later correction of deformity at the knee joint, because the foot has already been placed in a plantigrade position relative to the original deformity of the tibial mechanical axis. Therefore, in cases such as this, the patient may require revision for correct alignment of the hindfoot.[3]

PREOPERATIVE PLANNING

A thorough history and examination is critical in providing a diagnosis and outlining indications that will determine the direction of the operative procedure. It is important to review the anticipated outcome of the procedure with the patient so that a realistic goal can be met by both the patient and surgeon. The patient must understand that the time to recovery from this procedure, even with an optimal outcome, is long and challenging, and must not be taken lightly. Patients should be evaluated in a standing position to establish whether the foot is in a plantigrade position to determine the need for correction of angular relationships. The foot should also be evaluated in a non–weight-bearing position to evaluate range of motion and stability. Any osseous prominences or callosities should be noted. Observing the patient's gait can allow the surgeon to observe functional derangements that are causing symptoms. The inability to perform a single limb heel rise facilitates the diagnosis of posterior tibial tendon dysfunction. Severe hindfoot valgus is observed when excessive abduction of the forefoot produces a too-many-toes" sign. Radiographs of both the foot and ankle should be evaluated.

Evaluation of disorders at the knee joint must be taken into consideration. Patients with longstanding planovalgus deformity also present with lateral knee discomfort and arthritic changes. It is suggested that the patient address the knee deformity before undergoing correction of the foot so that the foot may be positioned plantigrade to the leg.

Ankle joint disorders and degeneration must be taken into consideration when preoperatively planning. A patient who displays both ankle and rearfoot joint degeneration may benefit more from a pantalar arthrodesis. Typically, this is performed in a staged process.

RADIOGRAPHIC EVALUATION

All patients should have weight-bearing radiographs of their feet and ankles: antero-posterior foot, lateral foot, and anteroposterior ankle views. Oblique foot and a mortise view may be taken as well to facilitate preoperative evaluation. Talar head uncovering is seen on anteroposterior view in patients with planovalgus deformity (**Fig. 2**). These patients also display divergence of the talocalcaneal angle on both the anteroposterior and lateral views. Conversely, these angles tend to be parallel or converge in patients with cavus foot type. The anteroposterior view of the ankle can be used to evaluate any degenerative joint disease, talar tilt, or to visualize calcaneal fibular impingement that is seen with flatfoot deformity.[5]

Other advanced imaging studies such as computed tomography, bone scanning, and magnetic resonance imaging are generally not required for preoperative evalua-tion. Advanced imaging may prove useful if there is suspicion of avascular necrosis of bone, or in instances in which posttraumatic primary arthrodesis in conjunction with open reduction and internal fixation is being undertaken. If there is a question of infection to bone, this may be confirmed with advanced imaging; however, arthrod-esis should not be performed when there is active infection.

SURGICAL TECHNIQUE

Preferably a tourniquet is placed around the upper calf region. Generous soft roll under-padding is placed around the undersurface of the tourniquet, particularly surrounding the course of the peroneal nerve as it wraps around the fibular head to impart adequate protection. This technique allows for the use of lower cuff pressures, typically around 250 mm Hg, compared with higher thigh tourniquets. Standard lower extremity surgical prep and draping may be used. The toes and forefoot may be covered using a surgical glove or iodine adhesive plastic to prevent contamination from debris from the toenails. Appropriate preoperative antibiotic therapy is advocated.[3]

Proper incisional placement is a key to allowing for sufficient anatomic exposure and ultimately proper reduction of the deformity. The 2-incisional approach is most commonly used; however, alternative single-incisional approaches may be used but do not impart the same degree of exposure.

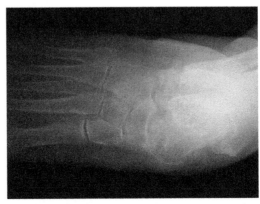

Fig. 2. Anterior posterior view flatfoot. Talar head uncovering may be visualized. Note the divergence of the talocalcaneal angle.

The lateral incision allows for exposure the subtalar, sinus tarsi, calcaneal cuboid, and lateral talonavicular joint articulations. The incision begins 1 cm distal to the tip of the lateral malleolus, extends along the lateral margin of the floor of the sinus tarsi, and ends along the base of the fourth metatarsal. Correct placement of this incisional line is parallel and between the course of the intermediate dorsal cutaneous and sural nerves. Occasionally, a communicating branch between these 2 nerves may be seen, and may be carefully resected if it will be traumatized during surgery.

Lateral dissection is typically initiated first. The peroneal tendons should be identified running along the lateral inferior aspect of the calcaneus and calcaneal cuboid articulation and retracted inferiorly. Next, the extensor digitorum brevis muscle belly is identified. The deep fascial, capsular, and periosteal tissues overlying the subtalar and calcaneal cuboid joint are opened simultaneously as 1 layer through and inverted-L–shaped flap. The flap is then reflected distally. There may be a large venous plexus along the distal extent of the extensor digitorum brevis muscle belly, so care should be taken to achieve proper hemostasis to prevent possible postoperative complications. The sinus tarsi may now be visualized (**Fig. 3**). The contents of the sinus tarsi are evacuated by using a hand rongeur or by placing a #15 blade along the osseous constraints of the talus and calcaneus and carefully moving the blade in a circular fashion. Care should be taken that all intertarsal ligaments are removed to allow the calcaneus to be reduced from its valgus position. Visualization of the posterior facet of the subtalar joint can now be made through the void in the sinus tarsi. A lamina spreader is then placed within the subtalar joint to allow wider exposure (**Fig. 4**).

Joint resection along the lateral extent of the foot is initiated through a technique referred to as contoured resection. This technique allows for complete removal of all cartilage and subchondral plate from the joint surfaces with an effort being made to maintain the anatomic contour. Maintaining the anatomic contour results in less shortening. The technique mainly uses hand instrumentation including curettes and osteotomes. Power instrumentation, such as a rotary burr, may be used; however, fine anatomic subtleties may be sacrificed. Power instrumentation must be used carefully because overuse also enhances thermal necrosis of bone. Once appropriate resection of the subtalar joint and calcaneal cuboid joints has been performed, the surgeon may move on to the medial dissection.

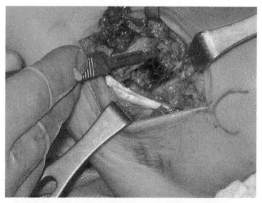

Fig. 3. Lateral surgical exposure. Note the peroneal tendon coursing below the calcaneocuboid joint. The extensor digitorum brevis belly is reflected distally. The sinus tarsi is visualized centrally. The subtalar plug (Hoke tonsil) may now be evacuated.

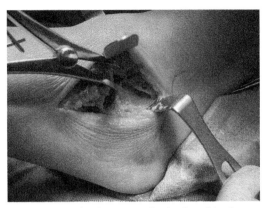

Fig. 4. Subtalar joint exposure. A laminar spreader is placed both anteriorly, for posterior exposure, and posteriorly, for anterior exposure in the subtalar joint for contoured resection of the facets.

The medial incision provides exposure of the talocalcaneal articulation, including the neck of the talus. The incision begins along the superior aspect of the medial malleolar articulation between the talus and the tibia in the ankle joint. The incision then courses distally across the prominence of the navicular and ends along the inferior margin of the navicular cuneiform joint. The incision is based medial to the tibialis anterior tendon.

Attention must be paid to avoiding the saphenous nerve and medial marginal vein. Several large communicating branches from the medial marginal vein may be encountered, as well as a network of vessels that lies just proximal to the talonavicular joint, and these should be properly identified and ligated or cauterized as dissection continues.

Care should be taken not to disrupt the distal course of the tibialis anterior tendon as it is identified at the level of the medial cuneiform. Reflection of the periosteal and capsular tissue is performed, allowing exposure to the talonavicular articulation. Subcapsular release along the overlying neck of the talus is performed until the ankle joint is visualized. At this point, it should be possible for the medial and lateral exposure to communicate with each other in the region overlying the neck of the talus. A malleable retractor may be placed in this region beneath the anterior neurovascular structures as they cross the ankle joint and enter the foot, imparting protection to them as joint resection is continued. Contoured resection of the talonavicular joint is performed. A lamina spreader may be used to facilitate exposure (**Fig. 5**).

If the patient has a rigid deformity, there may be limited mobilization of the subtalar joint with initial exposure, thus making resection within this joint difficult initially. In these instances, the surgeon may elect to resect the midtarsal joints first to afford greater soft tissue relaxation and facilitate entry into the subtalar joint. When resecting the midtarsal joints, it is best to begin at the talonavicular joint and then proceed to the calcaneocuboid joint.

Once the cartilage and subchondral plate have been resected, the bone begins to display a speckled red appearance, also described as a paprika sign, indicating appropriate preparation of the joint surfaces. The bone surfaces may then be further prepared by fenestrating with multiple small drill holes via a 0.62 K-wire or via fishscaling of the joint surfaces with an osteotome, which help to increase the vascularity and surface area, respectively, of the fusion sites.

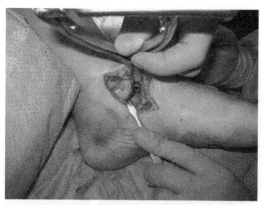

Fig. 5. Medial exposure. Medial dissection through the deep fascia is continued until the talar head is visualized. A laminar spreader is now used to facilitate exposure to the talonavicular joint for continued contoured resection.

The foot is then manipulated to achieve proper alignment for placement of provisional fixation by K-wires, Steinman pins, or guide wires from cannulated screwing systems. Achieving optimal positioning is critical to obtaining a plantigrade-type foot that is less susceptible to gait disturbances and adjacent joint development of arthritis. Fluoroscopy is used to confirm positioning and alignment. When positioning, the heel is placed vertical to the lower leg, the forefoot parallel to the hindfoot, and the first ray at the same level as the metatarsals. A calcaneal axial view is used to ensure that the long axis of the calcaneus is parallel to the mid-diaphyseal line of the distal tibia. The forefoot is positioned parallel to the hindfoot in both the frontal and transverse planes. The goal is a parallel rearfoot-to-leg relationship.[1] The Meary angle and Simon angle are evaluated to assess proper alignment in both the sagittal and transverse planes.

Once provisional fixation has been placed and appropriate alignment has been confirmed, rigid internal fixation may then be established. The subtalar joint is fixated through the use of either 1 or 2 6.5-mm diameter or greater partially threaded cancellous screws. The talonavicular and calcaneal cuboid joints are fixated using a combination of 4.0-mm or larger screws, staples, or miniplating systems. Washers may also be used in patients with poor bone stock. An alternative method of fixation is the use of external fixators, which may be used independently or combined with the use of internal fixation. External fixators allow for both static, as well as, dynamic compression. They are often helpful when performing a primary arthrodesis in a traumatic foot where purchase of internal fixation may not be possible (**Fig. 6**).

The wound is then irrigated and bone grafting is performed as necessary to fill any remaining osseous defects, particularly within the sinus tarsi region.

Closure of the surgical sites is performed in an anatomic fashion. The skin is closed using either suture or skin staples.

THE MEDIAL APPROACH TO TRIPLE ARTHRODESIS

A single incision for triple arthrodesis, although less common, may be used in a severe fixed valgus deformity. The approach is performed by making a single extensile incision that spans from behind the medial malleolus and extends distally toward the naviculocuneiform joint. Care must be taken that the incision remains dorsal to the

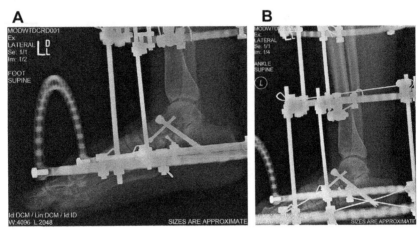

Fig. 6. (*A* and *B*) Adjunctive external fixation. External fixation at the surgeon's discretion may be used as an adjunct if internal fixation is not deemed adequate.

neurovascular bundle. The plane of dissection is between the tendons of the flexor hallucis longus and flexor digitorum longus. The tendon of the flexor hallucis longus is retracted inferiorly, thereby protecting the neurovascular bundle during joint resection.[6]

With this approach, resection of the talonavicular joint is initiated first. The talonavicular joint being the most prominent because of the severe abduction deformity present allows for easy identification and access to the joint surface. The middle facet along the head of the talus is visualized next. It should become possible to access the subtalar joint initially through the use of a curved osteotome, until a lamina spreader can placed within the joint to allow further exposure. Adequate visualization of the subtalar joint should now be possible to allow for appropriate joint resection. It is often preferable to remove a greater amount of bone from the medial aspect of the subtalar joint surface, because this allows for ease during realignment and correction of the valgus deformity. Removal of a wedge from the head of the navicular may be performed, allowing the foot to adduct around the transverse tarsal joint. This technique also shortens the medial column, allowing further correction of the valgus deformity. There is now more room for exposure to access the calcaneal cuboid joint. A guide pin may be placed across the transverse tarsal joint and verified via fluoroscopy to determine the exact location of the calcaneal cuboid joint. An osteotome is then used to cut across the calcaneal cuboid joint surfaces. The hindfoot is then aligned in a neutral position and fixation is placed. The midfoot is then passively pronated, adducted, and plantarflexed to achieve a plantigrade position, and fixation is placed across the talonavicular joint.[6]

ADJUNCTIVE PROCEDURES

Depending on the severity of the deformity to be corrected, it is common that the surgeon may need to perform another procedure in addition to the traditional triple arthrodesis. Adjunctive procedures include posterior muscle complex lengthening, posterior calcaneal osteotomies, lateral column lengthening, and bone grafting.

Equinus contracture of the posterior muscle complex is a commonly encountered finding. The patient must be evaluated using the Silfverskiold test before surgery to determine the appropriate procedure to allow for lengthening of the posterior muscle complex. The patient will undergo either a gastrocnemius lengthening or percutaneous Achilles tendon lengthening.[7,8] This is best performed at the start of the procedure to allow for appropriate laxity during repositioning and alignment for fixation.

A separate incision is needed when performing a calcaneal sliding osteotomy. This incision is performed before beginning exposure for the triple arthrodesis. This procedure allows for mechanical support of the ankle when there is failure of the posterior tibial tendon. The calcaneus is shifted approximately 10 to 12 mm medially. Temporary fixation is then placed across the osteotomy site into the body of the calcaneus. Following resection of the subtalar joint surfaces, a single screw may be used to fixate both the calcaneal osteotomy and subtalar joint.[9]

Lateral column lengthening may be performed through insertion of a bone wedge along the calcaneal cuboid joint. The bone wedge may be fixated in place, preferably with a small plate and screws, which allows the foot to be rotated out of supination and abduction about the midtarsal joint axis while limiting the amount of joint resection (**Fig. 7**). In a study by Horton and colleagues,[10] lateral column lengthening with triple arthrodesis was performed on 22 feet in 19 patients with severe planovalgus deformity. All patients achieved solid fusion in 12 weeks, with an average correction of the talus first metatarsal angle of 25° in both the anteroposterior and lateral planes.

Removal of bone wedges may be performed during the procedure to allow for further correction and reduction of the deformity in various planes. Sagittal plane correction is performed along the midtarsal joint axis as bone is resected. If a greater

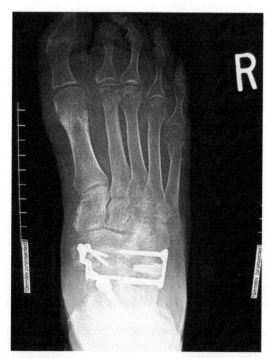

Fig. 7. Lateral column lengthening procedure. Anteroposterior radiograph depicts bone wedging to facilitate lengthening of the lateral column, which is done after resection of the calcaneocuboid joint articular surfaces and placed accordingly.

amount of bone is resected from the dorsal aspect of the joint, the patient's arch will effectively be lowered. Alternatively, if more bone is removed from the plantar aspect of the joint, the patient's arch will be raised. Abduction of the forefoot is performed as described earlier with a lateral column lengthening with insertion of bone graft. To achieve adduction of the forefoot, a medially based wedge of bone is resected from the midtarsal joint. Care must be taken not to remove too much navicular bone, because it will become difficult to place internal fixation.

POSTOPERATIVE MANAGEMENT

An initial postoperative Jones compression dressing is placed on the patient's lower extremity. Care is taken to be certain that the splint is in neutral position. It is the surgeon's preference whether or not a TLS drain is used. Typically, the patient is admitted to the hospital after surgery for pain management and observation. It is preferable for the patient to receive either a combined common peroneal and popliteal nerve block or an ankle block to aid in postoperative pain control. It is also important that the patient receives proper postoperative deep venous thrombosis prophylaxis. The lower extremity is to receive strict elevation and application of ice to control edema. At the first postoperative visit, if swelling is well controlled, a below-knee cast may be applied. The patient is to remain in a non–weight-bearing cast for 8 to 10 weeks. Crutches, a walker, or a wheelchair are used to assist the patient during this period. The patient may then be transitioned to a weight-bearing cam walker boot for an additional 2 to 3 weeks. Serial radiographs are required every 4 weeks. Physical therapy may be used following the patient's return to activity. Physical therapy facilitates strengthening and gait training.

COMPLICATIONS

As extensive as the procedure of a triple arthrodesis is, so is the potential for associated complications. The potential for these complications should be discussed with the patient when weighing the risks versus benefits of the procedure.

Among potential complications, nonunion is the most common. Although the rate of nonunion has improved in recent years with the advent of more rigid internal fixation, bone grafting, and improved surgical technique, nonunion rates in the literature have been noted to range from 5% to 10%.[3] The most common site for nonunion in triple arthrodesis has been found to be the talonavicular joint.[11] The use of bone grafting has helped to reduce the incidence of nonunion. Catanzariti and colleagues[5] described the use of bone grafting within the subtalar joint leading to extra-articular arthrodesis within the sinus tarsi. Risk factors leading to nonunion may include smoking, unstable internal fixation, inadequate resection of opposing surfaces, and nonadherence to postoperative non–weight-bearing instructions. A smoking cessation program is recommended in all patients who are smokers before undergoing the procedure.[2] If nonunion is observed 3 months after surgery, additional immobilization for another 4 to 6 weeks with follow-up radiographs is warranted. If osseous union is not observed by 6 months, revision surgery is recommended.

Malalignment can be avoided through careful intraoperative positioning of the foot. Care taken to avoid placing the foot in a supinated or varus position, because overloading of the lateral column will become intolerable to the patient. Undercorrection of the deformity may also lead to poor patient outcome. In a study by Maenpaa and colleagues,[11] 307 triple arthrodesis cases were reviewed, and malunion was the primary cause for revision surgery. Occasionally, malpositioning of the foot can be compensated for with the use of an orthotic after surgery; however, this condition usually requires surgical revision.

Nerve damage may occur as a result of the procedure. Most commonly, injury may occur to a branch of the superficial peroneal nerve. Care should be taken to ensure appropriate incision placement to avoid the course of the nerve. Anatomic dissection and retraction also facilitate avoidance of nerve injury. Occasionally, the sural nerve may be encountered because its course may arise slightly more superiorly. Care must be taken through anatomic dissection to avoid inadvertent laceration of the nerve.

Avascular necrosis is a rare complication, but must remain a concern. The predominant bone affected is the talus. Disruption of the blood supply may occur while accessing the subtalar joint, resecting a large portion of the talar head to increase correction of deformity, or excessive dissection of the talar neck while placing a screw from the talus down into the calcaneus.[9]

Wound healing problems may occur. Wound dehiscence may be secondary to poor hemostasis and development of postoperative hematoma. Some surgeons advocate the use of a drain after surgery. Poor tissue handling technique may predispose the skin to unnecessary trauma that may complicate healing as well. Wound healing complications are more likely to occur in patients who are smokers, diabetics, or those who are undergoing revision surgery and will have additional scar tissue development.

Painful hardware or hardware failure may be seen. Hardware is typically not removed unless it becomes intolerable to the patient. This situation is most likely to occur with screws placed retrograde across the subtalar joint.

DISCUSSION

Triple arthrodesis should only be considered when the symptoms and patient deformity are resistant to conservative therapy. The ultimate goal of the procedure for the patient is pain relief with restoration of malalignment. This result is obtained by establishing a plantigrade foot (**Fig. 8**). Patient selection and adherence to postoperative protocol is essential to obtaining an optimal result. Long-term results, with an average follow-up of 44 years, revealed that 95% of patients were satisfied with the procedure despite radiographic evidence of the development of proximal or distal joint degeneration.[2] However effective, triple arthrodesis is a challenging procedure for even the most skilled surgeon.

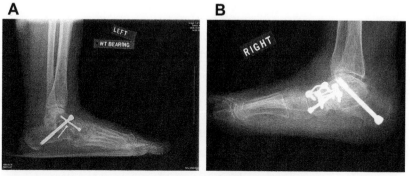

Fig. 8. (A and B) Plantigrade positioning after triple arthrodesis.

ACKNOWLEDGMENTS

The authors would like to acknowledge Joseph A. Mirarchi, BA, DPM, Rudy J. DeLuca, RPH, DPM, and David C. Kraatz, DPM for their contributions to this paper.

REFERENCES

1. Chang TJ. Triple arthrodesis. In: Master techniques in podiatric medicine and surgery: the foot and ankle. Philadelphia: Lippincott Williams & Wilkins; 2005. p. 377–94.
2. Thordarson DB. Foot and ankle. orthopedic surgery essentials. Philadelphia: Lippincott Williams & Wilkins; 2004. p. 213–5.
3. Wiss D. Talus-calcaneus-cuboid (triple) arthrodesis. In: Master techniques in orthopedic surgery. Philadelphia: Lippincott Williams & Wilkins; 2002. p. 401–24.
4. Wetmore RS, Drennan JC. Long-term results of triple arthrodesis in Charcot-Marie-tooth disease. J Bone Joint Surg 1989;71A:417–22.
5. Catanzariti AR, Mendicino RM, Saltrick KS, et al. Subtalar joint arthrodesis. J Am Podiatr Med Assoc 2005;95(1):34–41.
6. Myerson M. Triple arthrodesis. In: Reconstructive foot and ankle surgery. Philadelphia: Elsevier Saunders; 2005. p. 419–41.
7. Maskill MP, Loveland JD, Mendicino RW, et al. Triple arthrodesis for the adult-acquired flatfoot deformity. Clin Podiatr Med Surg 2007;24(4):765–78.
8. Ryerson EW. Arthrodesing operations on the feet. J Bone Joint Surg 1923;5:453–71.
9. Duncan JW, Lovell WW. Hoke triple arthrodesis. J Bone Joint Surg Am 1978;60(6):795–8.
10. Horton GA, Olney BW. Triple arthrodesis with lateral column lengthening for treatment of severe planovalgus deformity. Foot Ankle Int 1995;16(7):395–400.
11. Maenpaa H, Lehto MU, Belt EA. What went wrong in triple arthrodesis? An analysis of failures in 21 patients. Clin Orthop Relat Res 2001;391:218–23.

Ankle Arthrodesis

Steven F. Boc, DPM[a,b], Nathan D. Norem, DPM[c],*

KEYWORDS

• Ankle • Arthrodesis • Fusion • Tibiotalocalcaneal

Ankle arthrodesis was first described by Albert in 1879 as part of a knee and ankle fusion in a child suffering from palsy.[1] The early 1900s saw the use of arthrodesis in the ankle and foot for stabilization of paralysis secondary to polio. Then, in the 1950s, Charnely introduced an external fixator device for compression arthrodesis. His method was the first to use surgical hardware to place a compressive force across the arthrodesis site, thereby improving surgical outcomes. However, Charnely used a down to bone transverse incision at the level of the ankle joint, resulting in transection of tendons, nerves, and vascular structures with resulting sequelae.[2]

Building from Charnely's idea of compression across the osteotomy site, modern techniques for ankle arthrodesis now favor internal screw fixation, intramedullary nailing, arthroscopic joint preparation, plating, and improved external fixators. This resulting improvement in equipment technology and refinement of surgical technique have significantly improved fusion rates and decreased postoperative complications.

INDICATIONS

Painful arthrosis of the ankle joint with or without concurrent deformity is the primary indication for arthrodesis.[3,4] The typical candidate presents with a history of trauma, often involving articular damage to the ankle joint.[5] Specifically crushing injuries, comminuted fractures, and ankle sprains involving condylar cartilage injury are present. Other causes for ankle degeneration indicating arthrodesis may include failed implant, neoplasms, avascular necrosis, infection, Charcot, and congenital deformity.[6–9] Systemic arthritides, such as rheumatoid, show high correlations with ankle and subtalar deformities and degeneration. Michelson and colleagues[10] showed most rheumatoid patients experienced foot and ankle arthritis, 20% of whom have radiographic changes. Saltzman and colleagues[5] found 12% of patients in their study had arthritic ankles secondary to rheumatoid.

The authors have nothing to disclose.
[a] Podiatric Medicine and Surgery Residency Program, Drexel University College of Medicine/Hahnemann University Hospital, Philadelphia, PA 19107, USA
[b] Department of Surgery, Drexel University College of Medicine, Philadelphia, PA, USA
[c] Foot and Ankle Surgical Residency Program, Hahnemann University Hospital/Drexel University College of Medicine, Philadelphia, PA, USA
* Corresponding author. 235 North Broad Street, Suite 300, Philadelphia, PA 19107-1511.
E-mail address: nathannorem@gmail.com

Clin Podiatr Med Surg 29 (2012) 103–113
doi:10.1016/j.cpm.2011.10.005
0891-8422/12/$ – see front matter © 2012 Elsevier Inc. All rights reserved.

podiatric.theclinics.com

CONTRAINDICATIONS

When considering ankle arthrodesis, adequate soft tissue quality is of the utmost importance. Comorbidities including peripheral vascular disease, lymphedema, and venous stasis may prevent a patient from tolerating more involved tissue dissection and put the patient as risk for infection and amputation.[9,11,12] Smoking tobacco merits consideration because it has been shown to have a negative impact on bone fusion.[13] Complex lower extremity deformity with recurrence or progression may result in an unfavorable outcome. Other factors such as the patient's age, activity, quality of life, and surgical risk versus benefit need to be taken into consideration.

PREOPERATIVE ASSESSMENT

The initial clinical evaluation should determine any previous traumatic events, including sprains or fracture, because these are the most common cause of ankle arthritis.[2–4] Additional historical inquiry should screen for systemic illness including obesity, osteoporosis, gout, arthritis, infection, diabetes mellitus, neuropathy, and peripheral vascular disease. The patient's medications should be carefully reviewed because immunosuppressives are a standard therapy for inflammatory arthritides. Physical examination follows standard neurovascular testing and palpation for tender locations indicating concurrent disease. Biomechanical examination follows standard protocol with walking and static evaluation and special attention paid to the alignment of the rearfoot. This assessment should be a bilateral lower extremity examination, taking into account any existing deformity that may prevent a plantigrade foot. Sometimes the patient has an extremity or postural deformity that, on placing the ankle into normal alignment, inhibits a pain-free functional surgical outcome. The ankle may be put into a more neutral position for a forefoot valgus or greater than 5° valgus to compensate for a forefoot varus.[14]

Plain film radiographs may or may not show findings consistent with the clinical pain of which the patient is complaining.[15] However, often osteophytic formation, decreased joint space, and asymmetrical joint contour are hallmarks of an arthritic ankle.[16] In addition to the standard anterior posterior, mortise, and lateral views, long leg axial calcaneal views allow assessment of the hindfoot deformity (**Fig. 1**).[17] When considering surgical fusion one should seek out adjunctive imaging in the

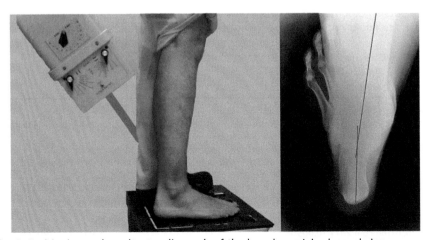

Fig. 1. Positioning and resultant radiograph of the long leg axial calcaneal view.

form of magnetic resonance imaging or computed tomography. These modalities allow greater examination of deformity, bone density, congruity, and retained hardware.[18] An invaluable addition to the standard computed tomography is volume rendering and shaded surface display three-dimensional reconstructions (**Fig. 2**). These technologies provide orientation of bone to overlying soft tissue and isolation of individual osseous structures, allowing greater visualization in significant deformities of the ankle joint and hindfoot and aiding in preoperative planning.[19,20]

SURGICAL TECHNIQUE

The preferred method at our institution for isolated ankle arthrodesis is the transfibular approach with or without fibular onlay graft. For combined talocalcaneal and tibiotalar arthrodesis, the intramedullary nail technique is used. These methods, in addition to endoscopic and various internal fixation techniques, are described.

Transfibular Approach Using Tripod Screw Technique

The patient is placed on the operative table in supine position with application of a thigh tourniquet and hip bump to align the knee and lower extremity. The lateral incision is made approximately 7 cm proximal to the ankle joint over the lateral fibula and is carried distally over the fibula, curving gently over the lateral aspect of the talus to a point approximately 1 cm distal to the tip of the fibula (**Fig. 3**). Dissection is then carried down through subcutaneous tissue to the level of the fibula; care should be taken to avoid the sural nerve and perforating peroneal arteries.[21] Deep dissection is made over the anterior ankle joint; the anterior tendon and neurovascular structures should be protected using a malleable retractor (**Fig. 4**). The surgeon now has the choice of either a transverse or an oblique osteotomy of the fibula. The oblique osteotomy allows repair of the fibula, whereas a transverse osteotomy may be used if a fibular onlay graft is desired.[14,22] The fibula is then reflected distally or removed (if removed it is transected longitudinally for use as an onlay graft) (**Fig. 5**). Depending on the desired positioning and deformity, the joint surfaces may be prepared as is, leaving the existing anatomic relationship, or planed with a saw to achieve the desired positioning. Cartilage is typically removed with a power burr and osteotome down to the level of bleeding, cancellous bone. Care must be taken to curette or osteotome any existing subchondral cystic structures. The medial malleolus cartilage can be removed via a curette through the lateral incision or a medial incision can be performed.[21,23–25]

A linear incision is made over the anterior medial malleolus and deepened down to the medial gutter/anterior ankle joint (**Fig. 6**). The saphenous nerve and vein must be

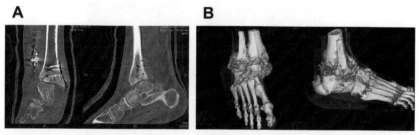

A   **B**

Fig. 2. (*A*) Computed tomography scan showing the visualization of retained hardware and degeneration of the ankle mortise. (*B*) Three-dimensional reconstruction of a significantly displaced ankle and subtalar joint.

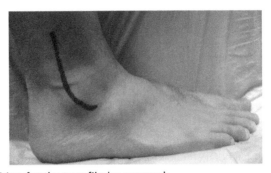

Fig. 3. Lateral incision for the transfibular approach.

identified and preserved during dissection. The anterior ankle capsule is then incised and reflected with an elevator, and resection of the cartilage can commence as described earlier. This approach also provides the option of a transmalleolar osteotomy of the tibia. The medial malleolus can be removed, allowing greater access for joint preparation and screw placement. All prepared joint surfaces are subchondral drilled with a 1.6-mm Kirschner wire.[21,23–25]

After adequate preparation of the joint, the knee/patella is palpated and marked by an assistant who holds the extremity in the correct orientation. The foot is then placed in 90° dorsiflexion (neutral) in the sagittal plane, 5° abduction in the transverse plane, a slight valgus in the frontal plane, and a posterior displacement of the foot relative to the tibia. The valgus positioning and subsequent eversion of the subtalar joint result in unlocking of the midtarsal joint, thereby allowing compensatory motion in the frontal and sagittal planes. The posterior displacement of the talus relative to the tibia allows for a shorter protrusion of the foot and eases transition to forefoot loading and toe off during gait. Position and apposition of the joint are viewed under intraoperative fluoroscopy.

Once the desired position/correction is achieved, temporary 1.6-mm Kirschner wires are driven to hold during insertion of the 3 6.5-mm cannulated screws.[14,21–25]

The first screw is inserted from the medial aspect either through the previously made incision or percutaneously if performing a strictly lateral approach. The entry point is posterior medial tibia to plantar lateral talar head. This home-run screw

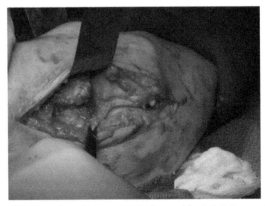

Fig. 4. Malleable retractor placed across anterior ankle joint to protect neurovascular structures and tendons.

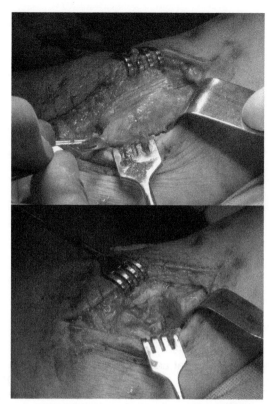

Fig. 5. Transverse cut is made through the fibula (*top*) and the fibula is removed (*bottom*).

compresses the talus against the tibia and pulls it slightly posterior. One must be careful of the posterior tibial tendon, especially if performing percutaneous insertion. The second screw is inserted proximally at the medial midline of the tibia and aimed distal toward the lateral process of the talus. Again this may be performed percutaneously. The third screw is inserted anterior lateral proximal tibia to posterior medial talus distally (**Fig. 7**). Typically the short 16-mm thread pattern is used for all 3 screws.[21,22,24]

When performed correctly, the orientation of the tripod screw technique provides both rotational and sagittal stability.[24] However, poor insertional orientation (placing screws predominately in 1 plane) may lead to rocking of the fusion site, thereby violating the rigid fixation principle of bone healing.[20,26,27] Some investigators have advocated the use of crossings screws with an anterior tibia talus plate to prevent any motion or rocking by providing a tension band or buttress construct.[24]

After final confirmation of the fusion site via intraoperative fluoroscopy, the fibular onlay graft is applied. The graft must be transected longitudinally to exposed cancellous bone. In addition, the tibia/talar side of the graft site must be power burred and/or osteototomed to the level of bleeding bone. Typical fixation involves 2 4.0-mm cannulated cancellous screws driven lateral to medial, with the proximal screw purchasing the tibia and the distal screw purchasing the talar body (**Fig. 8**). Crushed cancellous bone graft is often used to fill any remaining defects.[14,21,22,24,25]

The deep tissue layers are then carefully closed with absorbable suture, followed by a surgical drain and skin closure with nylon. The patient is placed into a dry sterile

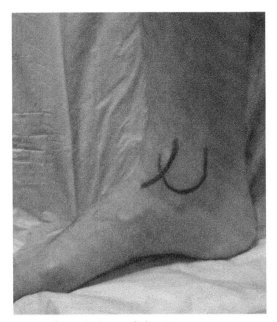

Fig. 6. Incision drawn over the anterior medial gutter.

gauze dressing and posterior splint and kept for observation. The drain is typically removed 48 to 72 hours later with application of a below-the-knee fiberglass cast before discharge. The postoperative course consists of 6 to 8 weeks of non–weight bearing in a below-the-knee cast, with interval cast changes every 2 weeks. Pending

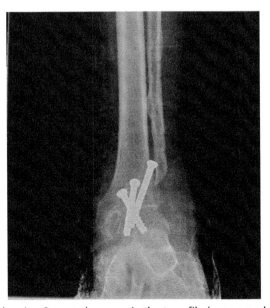

Fig. 7. The ankle showing 3 crossed screws via the transfibular approach.

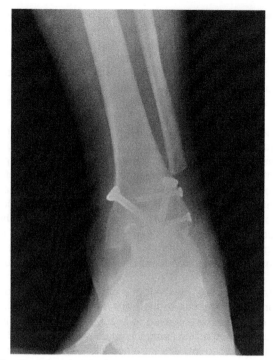

Fig. 8. Example of a fibular on lay graft with 2 crossed screws.

serial radiographic evidence of healing, the patient is then transitioned into a soft compressive cast and fracture walking boot, with protected weight bearing allowed for the next 4 weeks. At 12 weeks after surgery, the patient begins transitioning into normal shoe gear and may start physical therapy several weeks later depending on ambulatory status.

Intramedullary Nail Fixation

For patients with combined ankle and subtalar joint arthritis, the intramedullary rod or intramedullary nail is our procedure of choice. This form of fixation allows reduction and rigid fixation of significant talocalcaneal dislocations.[25,28,29]

The patient is placed on the operating table in the supine or lateral decubitus position. If placing supine, the use of a sterile, radiolucent extremity holder is recommended because posterior access to the foot during the procedure is difficult. The extremity is then scrubbed, prepared, and draped to the level of the knee.

Incision placement is similar to the crossed screws technique, with the cut beginning on the central lateral aspect of the fibular approximately 7 cm proximal to the joint line. The incision is then extended distally in a J fashion to the fourth metatarsal cuboid joint. Dissection is then carried deep to the level of the fibula and subtalar joint, with care taken to identify and preserve the sural nerve and perforating arteries. A transverse fibular osteotomy is then performed approximately 7 cm proximal from the tip of the fibula and the fibula is removed, exposing the ankle joint. Further dissection across the anterior aspect of the tibia is performed, protecting the anterior neurovascular structures.

A sagittal saw is used to resect the anterior and posterior aspects of the tibial pla-fond, creating a flat joint surface. The talus is also planed with a sagittal saw to a flat-tened or table-top shape. The reaming joint surfaces, including the medial malleolus, are curetted and osteotomed down to bleeding cancellous bone. Attention is then directed to the subtalar joint where joint resection down to bleeding bone is performed using the techniques described earlier. The posterior facet of the subtalar joint is the primary focus of joint preparation and is essential to successful fusion of the subtalar joint.[28]

At this stage, the patient is placed into alignment and viewed under intraoperative fluoroscopy for adequate joint congruity. In case of severe rearfoot displacement, significant portions of the talus may be absent and/or removed to properly align the calcaneus below the tibia. In these cases, the previously removed fibula may be cut and fashioned into a bicortical interpositional graft (**Fig. 9**).[11] Other acceptable grafts include femoral head allograft, talar body allograft, and iliac crest tricortical allograft.[30] The idea here is to preserve limb length and prevent shortening of the calcaneal talar distance. On most manufactures' nails this length is fixed and too much shortening may cause malalignment of the talar screw and/or a plantar grade nail. This situation causes difficulty inserting the posterior calcaneal screw and may cause it to be too far plantar.[29]

Under intraoperative fluoroscopy, the foot is placed in position under the tibia at 90° in the sagittal plane, 5° abduction in the transverse plane, and slight valgus in the frontal plane. The drill guide wire is used to fixate, and positioning is confirmed. The calcaneus and talus are then drilled along the guide wire along with the tibial metaphy-sis. A ball wire is then placed into the intramedullary canal and the position is again confirmed via fluoroscopy. Reaming and insertion of the nail then proceed per manu-facturer's guidelines.

In patients lacking a substantial talus or needing bone graft to maintain length, the use of the talar compression screw may be avoided and external compression with the jig can be used. After a final check of nail insertion length and position, any remaining bone void is filled with cancellous bone chips and/or demineralized bone matrix. The deep tissue layers are then closed and a drain is placed. The patient is placed into a Jones-style compressive dressing with a posterior fiberglass splint and admitted for observation.

The postoperative course consists of non–weight bearing in a below-the-knee fiber-glass cast for 6 to 8 weeks, with transition into a walking fracture boot pending evidence of radiographic healing. At 3 to 4 months, the patient is allowed to transition to normal shoe gear, and physical therapy is initiated if needed.

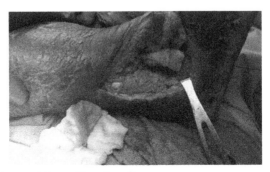

Fig. 9. Fibula used as an interpositional graft.

COMPLICATIONS

Postoperative complications of ankle arthrodesis include infection, numbness, hematoma, delayed union, malunion, and nonunion. Union rates of open ankle arthrodesis with internal fixation like the tripod screw technique have been reported in the 80% to 100% range.[31–33] Intramedullary nail tibiotalocalcaneal arthrodesis has similar reported fusion rates of 89% to 100% fusion at the ankle and slightly less success with concomitant subtalar fusion.[34,35]

Delayed union (defined as no evidence of radiographic healing after 3 months) is treated with continued below-the-knee casting, non–weight bearing, and an external bone stimulator. If the patient fails to respond and progress to a nonunion, additional surgical revision is required with aggressive resection of the fusion site and application of bone graft to prevent additional length loss. Malunion of the fusion site in plantar flexion, increased varus, or increased valgus typically induces increased stress on the compensatory motion of the midtarsal and subtalar joints.[36–39] The resulting degenerative changes may need further surgical intervention, especially in an isolated ankle fusion.

We have also experienced wound dehiscence leading to infection and subsequent osteomyelitis. This complication has been treated with removal of internal hardware and application of an external ring fixator during the usual 6-week intravenous antibiotics course. This procedure is followed by a revisional arthrodesis after confirming a negative set of bone cultures/pathology. If the patient previously had an isolated ankle fusion with screw fixation, we usually elect to use an intramedullary nail for the revision. In cases in which the intramedullary nail and space become infected, the nail is removed and an antibiotic spacer is inserted in conjunction with intravenous antibiotic therapy.[40]

SUMMARY

Ankle arthrodesis stands as a proven method for correction of moderate to severe deformity. Careful preoperative evaluation, imaging, and examination are crucial to obtaining an optimal functional result for the patient. The surgeon has numerous surgical options for obtaining fusion; the most popular and the most studied are crossed screws and/or plating. Additional techniques such as arthroscopic preparation and external fixators have provided satisfactory results in patients who may not tolerate an open approach. Deformity involving the subtalar joint can be addressed using an intramedullary nail to achieve tibiotalocalcaneal fusion.

REFERENCES

1. Albert E. Zur Resektion des Kniegelenkes. Wien Med Press 1879;20(5):705–8.
2. Charnley J. Compression arthrodesis of the ankle and shoulder. J Bone Joint Surg Br 1951;33(2):180–91.
3. Morgan CD, Henke JA, Bailey RW, et al. Long-term results of tibiotalar arthrodesis. J Bone Joint Surg Am 1985;67(4):546–50.
4. Takakura Y, Tanaka Y, Sugimoto K, et al. Long-term results of arthrodesis for osteoarthritis of the ankle. Clin Orthop Relat Res 1999;(361):178–85.
5. Saltzman CL, Salamon ML, Blanchard GM, et al. Epidemiology of ankle arthritis: report of a consecutive series of 639 patients from a tertiary orthopaedic center. Iowa Orthop J 2005;25:44–6.
6. Kitaoka HB, Romness DW. Arthrodesis for failed ankle arthroplasty. J Arthroplasty 1992;7(3):277–84.

7. Klouche S, El-Masri F, Graff W, et al. Arthrodesis with internal fixation of the infected ankle. J Foot Ankle Surg 2011;50(1):25–30.
8. Casadei R, Ruggieri P, Giuseppe T, et al. Ankle resection arthrodesis in patients with bone tumors. Foot Ankle Int 1994;15(5):242–9.
9. Ayoub MA. Ankle fractures in diabetic neuropathic arthropathy: can tibiotalar arthrodesis salvage the limb? J Bone Joint Surg Br 2008;90(7):906–14.
10. Michelson J, Easley M, Wigley FM, et al. Foot and ankle problems in rheumatoid arthritis. Foot Ankle Int 1994;15(11):608–13.
11. Nihal A, Gellman RE, Embil JM, et al. Ankle arthrodesis. Foot Ankle Surg 2008; 14(1):1–10.
12. Hirsch AT, Haskal ZJ, Hertzer NR, et al. ACC/AHA 2005 Practice Guidelines for the management of patients with peripheral arterial disease (lower extremity, renal, mesenteric, and abdominal aortic): a collaborative report from the American Association for Vascular Surgery/Society for Vascular Surgery, Society for Cardiovascular Angiography and Interventions, Society for Vascular Medicine and Biology, Society of Interventional Radiology, and the ACC/AHA Task Force on Practice Guidelines (Writing Committee to Develop Guidelines for the Management of Patients With Peripheral Arterial Disease): endorsed by the American Association of Cardiovascular and Pulmonary Rehabilitation; National Heart, Lung, and Blood Institute; Society for Vascular Nursing; TransAtlantic Inter-Society Consensus; and Vascular Disease Foundation. Circulation 2006;113(11):e463–654.
13. Greenhagen RM, Johnson AR, Bevilacqua NJ. Smoking cessation: the role of the foot and ankle surgeon. Foot Ankle Spec 2010;3(1):21–8.
14. McGlamry ED, Banks AS. McGlamry's comprehensive textbook of foot and ankle surgery. Philadelphia: Lippincott Williams & Wilkins; 2001.
15. Baan H, Drossaers-Bakker W, Dubbeldam R, et al. We should not forget the foot: relations between signs and symptoms, damage, and function in rheumatoid arthritis. Clin Rheumatol 2011;30(11):1475–9.
16. Thomas RH, Daniels TR. Ankle arthritis. J Bone Joint Surg Am 2003;85(5):923–36.
17. Saltzman CL, el-Khoury GY. The hindfoot alignment view. Foot Ankle Int 1995; 16(9):572–6.
18. Leffler S, Disler DG. MR imaging of tendon, ligament, and osseous abnormalities of the ankle and hindfoot. Radiol Clin North Am 2002;40(5):1147–70.
19. Morrison R, McCarty J, Cushing FR. Three-dimensional computerized tomography: a quantum leap in diagnostic imaging? J Foot Ankle Surg 1994;33(1): 72–6.
20. Choplin RH, Buckwalter KA, Rydberg J, et al. CT with 3D rendering of the tendons of the foot and ankle: technique, normal anatomy, and disease. Radiographics 2004;24(2):343–56.
21. Hendrickx RP, Kerkhoffs GM, Stufkens SA, et al. Ankle fusion using a 2-incision, 3-screw technique. Oper Orthop Traumatol 2011;23(2):131–40.
22. Schuberth JM, Ruch JA, Hansen ST Jr. The tripod fixation technique for ankle arthrodesis. J Foot Ankle Surg 2009;48(1):93–6.
23. Clissan DJ. The indications for inducing fusion at the ankle joint by operation; with description of two successful techniques. Aust N Z J Surg 1949;19(1): 64–71.
24. Ogilvie-Harris DJ, Fitsialos D, Hedman TP. Arthrodesis of the ankle. A comparison of two versus three screw fixation in a crossed configuration. Clin Orthop Relat Res 1994;(304):195–9.
25. Chang TJ. The foot and ankle. Philadelphia: Lippincott Williams & Wilkins; 2005.
26. Digby JM. Principles and practice of AO. NATNEWS 1985;22(Suppl 2):8–10.

27. Dohm MP, Benjamin JB, Harrison J, et al. A biomechanical evaluation of three forms of internal fixation used in ankle arthrodesis. Foot Ankle Int 1994;15(6): 297–300.
28. Myerson MS, Alvarez RG, Lam PW. Tibiocalcaneal arthrodesis for the management of severe ankle and hindfoot deformities. Foot Ankle Int 2000;21(8):643–50.
29. Klos K, Drechsel T, Gras F, et al. The use of a retrograde fixed-angle intramedullary nail for tibiocalcaneal arthrodesis after severe loss of the talus. Strategies Trauma Limb Reconstr 2009;4(2):95–102.
30. Cuttica DJ, Hyer CF. Femoral head allograft for tibiotalocalcaneal fusion using a cup and cone reamer technique. J Foot Ankle Surg 2011;50(1):126–9.
31. Perlman MH, Thordarson DB. Ankle fusion in a high risk population: an assessment of nonunion risk factors. Foot Ankle Int 1999;20(8):491–6.
32. Takenouchi K, Morishita M, Saitoh K, et al. Long-term results of ankle arthrodesis using an intramedullary nail with fins in patients with rheumatoid arthritis hindfoot deformity. J Nippon Med Sch 2009;76(5):240–6.
33. Scranton PE Jr. Use of internal compression in arthrodesis of the ankle. J Bone Joint Surg Am 1985;67(4):550–5.
34. Budnar VM, Hepple S, Harries WG, et al. Tibiotalocalcaneal arthrodesis with a curved, interlocking, intramedullary nail. Foot Ankle Int 2010;31(12):1085–92.
35. Boer R, Mader K, Pennig D, et al. Tibiotalocalcaneal arthrodesis using a reamed retrograde locking nail. Clin Orthop Relat Res 2007;463:151–6.
36. Mazur JM, Schwartz E, Simon SR. Ankle arthrodesis. Long-term follow-up with gait analysis. J Bone Joint Surg Am 1979;61(7):964–75.
37. Abdo RV, Wasilewski SA. Ankle arthrodesis: a long-term study. Foot Ankle 1992; 13(6):307–12.
38. Coester LM, Saltzman CL, Leupold J, et al. Long-term results following ankle arthrodesis for post-traumatic arthritis. J Bone Joint Surg Am 2001;83(2):219–28.
39. Jackson A, Glasgow M. Tarsal hypermobility after ankle fusion–fact or fiction? J Bone Joint Surg Br 1979;61(4):470–3.
40. Howell WR, Goulston C. Osteomyelitis: an update for hospitalists. Hosp Pract (Minneap) 2011;39(1):153–60.

Salvage Arthrodesis for Charcot Arthropathy

Panagiotis Panagakos, DPM[a], Nathan Ullom, DPM[b], Steven F. Boc, DPM[c],*

KEYWORDS

- Arthrodesis • Charcot • Limb salvage • External fixation
- Ulceration

EPIDEMIOLOGY

Charcot osteoarthropathy, also known as *neuropathic osteoarthropathy*, is a syndrome that results in the destruction of single or multiple joints leading to permanent joint deformity.[1] Joint changes as a result of neuropathic change were first described by Musgrave in 1703.[1] Most commonly credited with modern day definition of this condition is Jean Marie Charcot[2] for his 1868 analysis of neuropathic osteoarthropathy in patients with tabes dorsalis.

Currently, Charcot osteoarthropathy is most commonly associated with diabetes mellitus as the primary origin, but has been attributed to multiple conditions. Charcot osteoarthropathy has also been reported in connection with infection, spinal or peripheral nerve injury, alcoholism, trauma, cerebral palsy, syphilis, spina bifida, and multiple other medical disorders.[2] The identifying characteristic commonly shared among these conditions is significant decrease or loss of pain sensation to the area in question. In addition to neuropathy, previous authors suggest the presence of several other factors that may play contributing roles in the Charcot foot, including trauma, metabolic factors, arteriovenous shunting abnormalities, and absence of occlusive arterial disease.[3]

Historically, this condition is reported to affect a very small population, namely only 0.2% of the diabetic population, with a higher incidence reported among the diabetic population previously diagnosed with peripheral neuropathy.[2] Studies suggest that

The authors have nothing to disclose.

[a] Foot and Ankle Care Associates, LLC, Hahnemann University Hospital, Overlook Hospital, 612 West Fingerboard Road, Staten Island, NY 10305, USA
[b] Department of Podiatric Medical Education, Hahnemann University Hospital, 230 North Broad Street, Philadelphia, PA 19102, USA
[c] Podiatric Medicine and Surgery, Department of Surgery, Drexel College of Medicine, Hahnemann University Hospital, 235 North Broad Street, Philadelphia, PA 19107, USA
* Corresponding author.
E-mail address: Sfbocdpm1@comcast.net

Clin Podiatr Med Surg 29 (2012) 115–135
doi:10.1016/j.cpm.2011.10.001   **podiatric.theclinics.com**
0891-8422/12/$ – see front matter © 2012 Elsevier Inc. All rights reserved.

a significant number of Charcot cases go undiagnosed because of lack of clinical recognition by physicians, leading to more severe deformity in this patient population.[4,5] Early and accurate diagnosis of acute Charcot osteoarthropathy is of extreme importance in the clinical management of this condition.[5]

DIAGNOSIS/IMAGING

Diagnosing acute Charcot can be difficult. Patients typically present with significant localized edema, erythema, and warmth in the affected limb compared with the contralateral limb. Because of the common trio of symptoms on presentation, patients are often misdiagnosed with cellulitis, gout, or deep venous thrombosis.[6] Misdiagnosis of Charcot can lead to patients following incorrect treatment protocol, including antibiotic therapy; the absence of an offloading program, resulting in increased deforming forces on the limb; and even unnecessary amputations. An increased suspicion for Charcot is essential among the neuropathic diabetic population presenting with the aforementioned symptoms. Pedal pulses are typically present in patients with Charcot foot, because concomitant peripheral arterial disease is uncommon.[6] Patients with advanced Charcot or a previous history of the condition may present with an already deformed foot type. These patients commonly present with a rocker-bottom foot and are often affected by ulcerations plantarly.

Charcot osteoarthropathy primarily should be diagnosed clinically, but then plain film radiographs are useful in staging the condition and following its progression. The Charcot foot was originally classified radiographically by Eichenholtz[7] in 1966, who described three distinct developmental stages. Stage 1 is described as subchondral fragmentation and referred to as the *development stage*. Stage 2 is known as the *coalescence stage*, with absorption of small debris and fusing of larger fragments of bone, with notable sclerosis at both the proximal and distal aspect of the previously fragmented bone. Stage 3 is referred to as the *reconstructive phase*, with remodeling of the previously fragmented and recoalesced bone. Yu and Hudson[8] added a stage 0 to the Eichenholtz system for patients with diabetes, adding clinical signs of inflammation and trauma to the foot before radiographic evidence of the condition is noted.

A five-stage classification system was proposed by Sella and Baratte[9] in 1999. Stage 0 was defined as a clinical diagnosis with lack of radiographic evidence. Stage 1 included clinical findings and localized osteopenia, diastases, and cyst formation visualized on plain film radiograph. Stage 2 was defined as involving the presence of joint subluxation. Stage 3 involved significant collapse of the medial arch of the foot. Stage 4 was described as radiographic evidence of boney fusion with notable sclerosis in the areas of previously fragmented bone. An additional classification system that identifies specific joint involvement was described by Sanders and Frykberg,[10] which is helpful in identifying a specific location of involvement in the foot.[9]

Multiple imaging studies can be used in conjunction with or in addition to plain film radiograph. Triphasic bone scan has been historically used as a tool in identifying Charcot osteoarthropathy, although its usefulness is currently debated, because it is a nonspecific study and does not differentiate between Charcot osteoarthropathy and osteomyelitis.[11] More recently, use of a white blood cell–labeled bone scan has been proposed because of its ability to exclude osteomyelitis as a differential diagnosis, and is considered by many as the gold standard for differentiation.[11] MRI is also used by many physicians to differentiate Charcot from osteomyelitis, although widespread debate exists as to its ability to do so. Despite the fact that it is a poor tool for differentiation, some describe it as the gold standard for evaluating extent of involvement of either process.[11] The use of imaging studies to correlate a clinical diagnosis of Charcot osteoarthropathy and to evaluate progression of the condition can prove useful when assessing a treatment protocol for a patient.

MEDICAL TREATMENT

The widely accepted initial treatment protocol after diagnosis of acute Charcot osteo-arthropathy is complete offloading of the extremity with total contact casting, and local wound care for any ulceration.[12] Offloading the affected extremity avoids any deform-ing weight-bearing forces placed on the foot. The recommendation is for patients to remain non–weight-bearing in a total contact cast until all clinical and radiographic evidence of acute Charcot osteoarthropathy has dissipated, with the average length of casting reported as between 3 and 4.5 months.[13]

Pharmacologic intervention in the treatment of Charcot osteoarthropathy has recently been proposed to inhibit osteoclastic activation and excessive inflammatory response.[12] Bisphosphonates used in antiresorptive therapy have been shown in randomized trials to have a positive effect in patients with acute Charcot, helping to decrease foot temperature, with a decrease in bone turnover markers and no notable side effects.[14] The use of pharmacologic modalities as an adjunct to offloading therapy in the treatment of the Charcot foot is promising but currently lacking long-term large-scale studies to prove its efficacy.

OPERATIVE CONSIDERATIONS

Patients with Charcot are high-risk and usually present with multiple comorbidities. Before surgery, several tests and consultations must be performed to evaluate the patient's potential for healing and surviving the complex surgery. When a patient with Charcot who requires surgery presents to the authors' facility, a thorough history and physical examination are immediately performed. Foot, ankle, and leg radio-graphs and advanced imaging, such as CT scans or MRI, are necessary for surgical planning. The patient is then sent for noninvasive vascular studies. If vascular insuffi-ciency is present, then a revascularization procedure might be necessary. Medical clearance is a necessity. These patients usually require cardiology, nephrology, endo-crinology, or vascular clearance. Treatment of patients with Charcot should always be a team approach, with all providers understanding what each surgery entails. Stan-dard blood values are assessed and hemoglobin A1c, prealbumin, and albumin levels determined. Once a patient is in the operating room, appropriate antibiotics are administered. A thigh tourniquet is always used by the authors. After completion of the procedure, drains are always inserted and the patient is always admitted for obser-vation, deep vein thrombosis prophylaxis, and necessary medical care. When patients are stable for discharge, they are evaluated by the hospital's physical rehabilitation team and recommendations are made for home or a rehabilitation facility. After discharge from the hospital, the patient is followed in the authors' facilities at least once weekly for the first 3 months and once monthly thereafter for observation. Patient selection is very important, and proper medical care, from planning to discharge to follow-up, is a necessity for successful limb salvage in these patients and to limit the occurrences of lower limb amputations.

MIDFOOT ARTHRODESIS

Fracture-dislocation of the midfoot with collapse of the longitudinal arch is common in patients with neuropathic arthropathy of the foot. Patients with this midfoot collapse often have a rocker-bottom deformity that can lead to ulceration and osteomyelitis.

Midfoot fusion in these patients is a salvage procedure that can prevent ulceration and infection, therefore preserving the limb. Many techniques have been described in the literature for midtarsal fusion of the Charcot foot, all with its own advantages and disadvantages. The authors' indications for Charcot midfoot arthrodesis are:

- Any Charcot midfoot joint with collapse at the tarsometatarsal joints or rocker-bottom deformity that can lead to ulceration
- Any unstable Charcot midfoot joint for which conservative treatment has failed
- Recurrent ulceration from gross deformity
- Any progressive deformity of the Charcot midfoot with preulcerative lesion
- Any stable deformity with ulceration or preulcerative lesion.

The authors have noticed that when they follow these indications for salvage arthrodesis, the success of limb salvage increases through decreasing the rate of ulcer formation. The operative goal of any surgical procedure is to establish a stable plantigrade foot that can be fitted in a custom molded shoe or device, and to prevent ulceration. Contraindications to performing this procedure are the presence of bone infection, poor vascular supply, known poor patient compliance, poor nutritional status, or elevated or abnormal laboratory values that indicate poor wound healing. When treated with simple ostectomy, midfoot ulcers beneath the lateral column have a higher incidence of reulceration than those beneath the medial column. Therefore, lateral midfoot ulcers associated with Charcot deformity should be treated with arthrodesis.[15] Hamilton and Ford[16] stated that if bony resection of a midfoot prominence leaves an unstable structure, then progression of the rocker-bottom deformity and recurrent ulceration are likely. This article's authors strongly discourage and rarely perform simple ostectomies of the midfoot. They believe in correcting the deformity to prevent any future recurrences, and routinely perform a midfoot wedge osteotomy (**Fig. 1**). This osteotomy can correct deformities in the transverse and sagittal plane.

Some controversy exists in the literature regarding the appropriate timing of surgery. Some authors advocate performing the fusion procedure while in the acute stage, whereas others prefer waiting until the later stages of the Charcot process. Simon and colleagues[17] evaluated the use of arthrodesis of the tarsometatarsal area for the treatment of Eichenholtz stage 1 Charcot arthropathy. All 14 arthrodesis procedures were successful, resulting in anatomic alignment and clinical union. No patients had immediate or long-term complications, and none reported ulceration after the operation. Before this study, it was accepted that all fusions in a Charcot foot should wait until Eichenholtz stage 2 or 3 because performing the procedure earlier would lead to poor outcomes and further fragmentation and bony destruction. This study showed that fusing in stage 1 is easier because no gross deformity is present and excessive bony work is not necessary. The authors postulated that operating in the early stage did not seem to lengthen healing time and in fact may have expedited the reversal of the destructive process.

In another study, Roukis and colleagues[18] treated eight unstable Eichenholtz stage 1 diabetic Charcot foot deformities using open reduction internal fixation, immobilization in a non–weight-bearing cast for 8 to 10 weeks, and then a total-contact weight-bearing cast for 2 to 7 months. These feet remain stable and free from ulceration at a mean of 28 months.[18]

Studies have supported performing arthrodesis in Eichenholtz stage 2 and 3 Charcot feet with good results. Papa and colleagues[18,19] reviewed 29 patients who had osseous prominences with instability, performed an arthrodesis with open reduction internal fixation, then cast immobilization and finally custom ankle foot orthoses were used. At a mean of 5 months, 19 patients (66%) developed a solid arthrodesis,

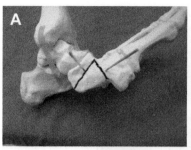
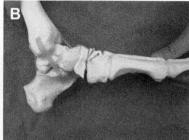
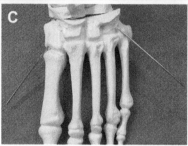

Fig. 1. (*A*) Midfoot biplanar wedge resection with converging guide wires for rocker-bottom deformity. (*B*) Removal of wedge and satisfactory bony apposition for midfoot fusion. (*C*) Provisional fixation with K-wires or guide wires from screw set.

10 patients developed a pseudoarthrosis, and 7 were stable. None of the patients treated who developed a solid arthrodesis or stable pseudoarthrosis broke down during the follow-up period of 43 months.

Early and Hansen[20] reviewed 21 feet with Eichenholtz stage 2 and 3 diabetic Charcot foot and osseous deformities with instability. They performed arthrodesis with open reduction internal fixation, tendo-achilles lengthening, cast immobilization, and wheelchair use. At a mean of 28 months, 18 feet (86%) had been treated successfully.

The authors have performed arthrodesis of the medial column and the entire midfoot complex with open reduction internal fixation in both the early and late stages of the Charcot process. They prefer to wait and use open reduction internal fixation in the late stages in additional to external fixation, and solely use external fixation in the early stages of the process. They believe it is difficult to perform an open reduction internal fixation in the acute Charcot process because of edema, obliteration of the soft tissue planes, and the soft fragmented bone. One can easily gouge excessive bone while resecting cartilage and debris from the joint surfaces because of lack of strength of the bony structures. Apposition of bony surfaces could potentially become more difficult. The authors treated an acute Charcot midfoot (**Fig. 2**) initially with external fixation, and soon after the patient experienced what is known as "cage rage" and the external fixator was removed. After removal, a medial column fusion was performed with a "superconstruct" plate, specifically designed for Charcot reconstructions. The patient progressed to a solid fusion, which is evident on postoperative advanced imaging, without complications. She is now ambulating in custom molded ankle foot orthoses and diabetic shoes. In this one case, the authors were able to achieve a solid fusion of an acute Charcot foot and prevent further progression of deformity.

The authors have used various techniques to achieve midfoot fusion in a Charcot foot. Fusion can be accomplished through internal fixation, external fixation, or a combination of both. They usually advocate a combination of internal and external

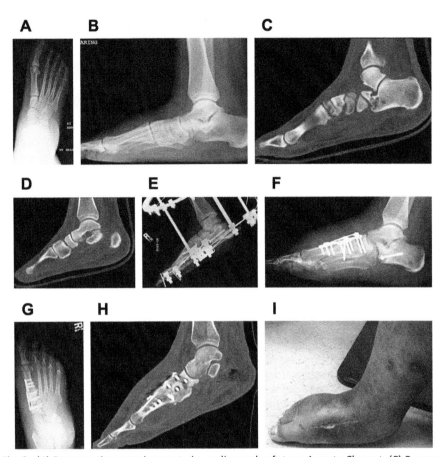

Fig. 2. (A) Preoperative anterior-posterior radiograph of stage 1 acute Charcot. (B) Preoperative lateral radiograph of stage 1 acute Charcot with soft tissue edema and the beginning of medial column collapse. (C) Preoperative CT scan showing anterior calcaneal fracture. (D) Preoperative CT scan showing slight navicular-cuneiform fault. (E) Application of external fixation and open reduction internal fixation of acute Charcot calcaneal fracture. (F) Removal of external fixation from "cage rage," and application of superconstruct for medial column fusion for acute Charcot. (G) Postoperative anteroposterior radiograph of medial column fusion for acute Charcot. (H) Postoperative CT scan demonstrating solid fusion of medial column for acute stage 1 Charcot. (I) Stable plantigrade foot status post medial column fusion of acute Charcot with a superconstruct plate. A minor wound is present over the surgical site, which healed without incident.

fixation devices to achieve an adequate fusion of the Charcot foot (**Fig. 3**). A recent technique described in the literature is beaming for midfoot arthrodesis. Beaming uses axial intramedullary large-diameter screws to realign the medial and lateral columns. Rooney and colleagues[21] introduced a technique of axial intramedullary fixation of the medial and lateral columns using long intramedullary screws. Assal and Stern[22] used a medial column intramedullary screw in 15 patients with Charcot with rocker-bottom deformity, 13 of whom had a plantar ulceration. All the patients underwent realignment with arthrodesis. At a mean of 42 months' follow-up, 14 patients were able to walk and no recurrent ulcers were seen. The investigators stated that a key advantage to using axial intramedullary fixation is that much less

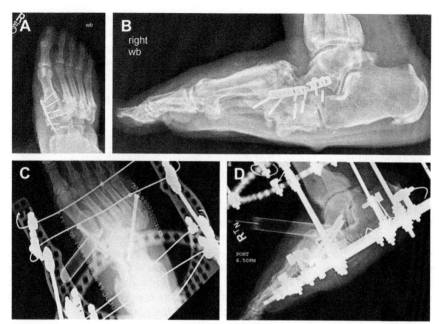

Fig. 3. (A) Anteroposterior radiograph with unstable Charcot midfoot with hardware failure. (B) Lateral radiograph showing unstable Charcot midfoot deformity with failed hardware and preulcerative lesion on plantar aspect. (C) Application of internal and external fixation after wedge resection for midfoot Charcot. (D) Application of internal and external fixation for Charcot midfoot after wedge resection. A plantigrade foot has been created with elimination of deformity.

dissection is required to insert the screw than to place a plate. They state that this technique prevents vascular compromise to the bone and decreases the rate of wound complications.

Sammarco and colleagues[23] retrospectively reviewed 22 patients who underwent beaming of the medial column for Charcot reconstruction. At an average of 52 months' follow-up, complete osseous union was seen in 16 patients; five partial unions were seen in which a single joint did not unite in an otherwise stable foot, and only one nonunion was seen, with recurrence of deformity. All the patients returned to an independent functional ambulatory status within 9.5 months.

Grant and colleagues[24] explained that beams behave like reinforcement rods, in the same manner that steel rebar serves to reinforce concrete. The beam acts to share the load with the bones, ligaments, and joints of the foot, thereby decreasing the sum of the bending forces on the bone through accepting axial forces of compression and tension sustained by the entire column. Therefore, the load of weight-bearing is distributed and shared with the intramedullary fixation rather than the bone receiving all the forces, helping to maintain anatomic alignment. The investigators state that beaming the medial and lateral columns seems to be the key to the durability of the hindfoot and LisFranc Charcot foot repairs. They reviewed 71 Charcot reconstructions that underwent beaming of the medial and lateral columns. In their retrospective study, they found significant improvement in preoperative and postoperative radiographic measurements, including Meary's angle and the calcaneal inclination, tarsometatarsal, talonavicular, and calcaneocuboid angles.

Other new advances in the treatment of midfoot fusion for Charcot arthropathy are the use of superconstruct locking plates. These relatively new plate designs span the entire length of the medial column, providing rigid stability and good anatomic alignment. Sammarco[25] described the four criteria necessary for hardware to be considered a superconstruct:

1. Fusion is extended beyond the zone of injury to include joints that are not affected, to improve fixation
2. Bone resection is performed to shorten the skeleton to allow for adequate reduction of the deformity without tension on the soft tissues
3. The strongest device is used that can be tolerated by the soft tissue
4. The devices are applied in a position that optimizes their mechanical function.

The authors have used these devices for midfoot arthrodesis with good results. The authors usually place them on the dorsomedial aspect of the medial column, which provides a good mechanical advantage. They avoid using plantar plates, which optimally are the best, because of the tension side being on the plantar surface. They feel that excessive dissection is needed to apply a plantar plate, and is anatomically challenging. One must be careful in selecting the appropriate patient when using these specialized plates. They are larger and thicker than conventional plates. Enough soft tissue envelope must be present to close over the construct. The authors have noticed some postoperative wound complications and plate exposures through the patients' skin when using these devices. For this reason, their preferred method of fixating a midfoot arthrodesis for Charcot collapse is the beaming technique of the medial and lateral columns, or using locking plates placed on the dorsomedial surface of the medial column in combination with external fixation (**Fig. 4**). Zonno and Myerson[26] stated that locking plates provide fixed-angle stability and have been shown to be four times stronger than conventional plates. They also provide improved fixation in osteoporotic bone. Locking plates preserve the periosteal blood supply and may assist in healing. These qualities make them ideal for use in Charcot foot reconstruction (**Fig. 5**).

For acute Eichenholtz stage 1 Charcot midfoot deformities, the authors prefer to use an external fixator until coalescence of bony structures is evident on radiographs and decreased edema and temperature of the affected limb is clinically apparent. Using external fixation for arthrodesis is not a new concept. It allows for micromotion to occur through fracture and joint dislocation areas, which can facilitate arthrodesis by compressing fragments or joint areas with arthropathy.[27] The authors believe in stabilizing the acute Charcot process, and prevent further bony destruction and deformity through applying an external fixator at this stage. They also prefer to use external fixation when an ulceration with or without infection is present in the acute phase of Charcot requiring deformity correction, or for an acute fracture in a patient with neuropathy. Because bone is soft and hyperemic during the acute phase of Charcot arthropathy, internal fixation often fails. Compared with internal fixation, small pins tensioned to a ring construct across the foot and ankle depend less on hard bone.[16] When midfoot osteomyelitis is present, the external fixator can be used to achieve a septic fusion or stabilize the remaining hindfoot bones.

The choice of external fixator depends on the surgeon's preference. In most cases the authors use a neutral three-ring design, which includes two tibial rings attached to a footplate (**Fig. 6**). The external fixator is applied after correction of the deformity has been accomplished. The authors measure the size of the leg and ankle preoperatively and prebuild their external fixator constructs, which makes them available for

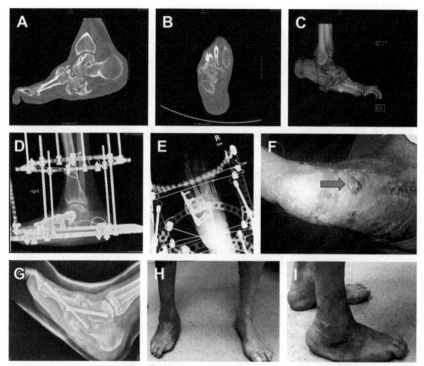

Fig. 4. (A) CT scan of stage 3 Charcot deformity with plantarly displaced cuboid. (B) CT scan showing midfoot Charcot changes. (C) Three-dimensional CT reconstruction showing rocker-bottom deformity with plantarly displaced cuboid. (D) Status post midfoot wedge osteotomy with superconstruct and external fixator application. (E) Status post Charcot reconstruction anteroposterior radiograph. (F) Exposed distal aspect of medial column superconstruct plate. (G) Status post removal of medial column plate. Beaming of medial and lateral columns. (H) Postoperative appearance at 1 year. (I) Postoperative appearance at 1 year.

immediate use in the operating room. Sterile towels are placed beneath the leg while applying the frame construct to accommodate for postoperative edema. Two olive wires are placed and tensioned on each tibial ring, two are inserted into the calcaneus, and two are placed crossing the metatarsals, which are appropriately tensioned. This technique creates the authors' basic three-ring frame construct. In a prospective study, Pinzur[28] used a similar neutral three-ring fixator for 26 morbidly obese patients with nonplantigrade Charcot midfoot deformity with ulceration. Fourteen feet had underlying wounds with osteomyelitis. At a minimum of 1-year follow-up, 24 of 26 feet were ulcer-free and infection-free and able to ambulate with custom diabetic shoes and orthoses. Pinzur concluded that morbidly obese patients with Charcot deformity and severe comorbidities can achieve correction of midfoot deformity after operative correction of the deformity and maintenance of that correction with a neutrally applied external fixator.

Other more-complicated external fixators can be designed for midfoot or tarsal fusion. An external fixator can bridge the arthrodesis site and neutralize stress. A multi-planar external fixation construct alone can provide adequate interfragmentary stabilization. This may be accomplished through the use of a bent-wire technique.[15] Grant and colleagues[29] concluded that the bent-wire technique increases the vector

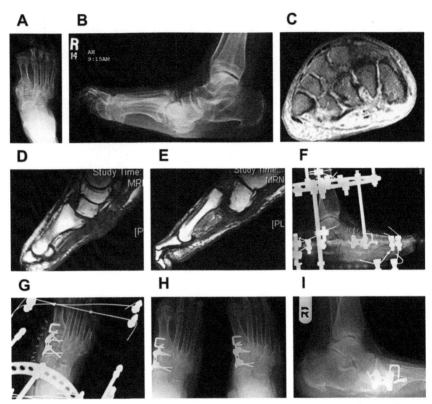

Fig. 5. (*A*) Preoperative anterior-posterior radiograph showing Stage 3 Charcot foot with dislocation at the tarsometatarsal joint. (*B*) Preoperative lateral radiograph of stage 3 Charcot showing rocker-bottom deformity. (*C*) Coronal section MRI showing dislocation at the tarsometatarsal joint. (*D*) Sagittal MRI showing rocker-bottom deformity. (*E*) Sagittal MRI showing rocker-bottom deformity of the lateral column. (*F*) Postoperative internal and external fixation combination. (*G*) Postoperative internal and external fixation combination. (*H*) Radiograph showing status 4 years after Charcot reconstruction. (*I*) Radiograph showing status 4 years after Charcot reconstruction with stable plantigrade foot.

forces of compression to create an apparent synergy between the internal and external forces, resulting in greater stability and interfragmentary compression at the fusion site.

The authors have used to the bent-wire technique to achieve uniform compression across an arthrodesis site for Charcot midfoot deformities with good predictable outcomes. In one case, a modified miter external fixator was applied to a Charcot foot with an infected plantar ulceration (**Fig. 7**). The transosseous wire is inserted distal to the arthrodesis site. The bent wire is attached proximal to where it emerged on the external fixator. At this point the wire is bent back at the same time using two wrenches, a technique that is usually referred to as *Russianing the wires*. Other more complex frames exist, including the Taylor Spatial Frame external fixation system (Smith & Nephew, Memphis, TN, USA) and the Adam Frame (Imed Surgical LLC, Lyndhurst, NJ, USA), which consist of struts attached to rings and are able to correct extremity deformities with computer-assisted programs. These devices can be difficult to apply, and good knowledge of the computer software is mandatory to achieve an adequate result.

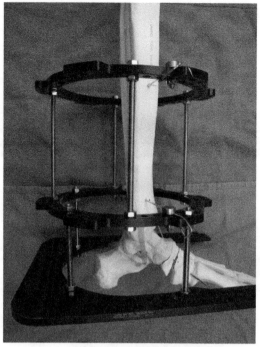

Fig. 6. Application of a neutral three-ring external fixator.

With all Charcot surgical reconstructions, it is important to address the equinus deformity. The negative effects of equinus have been well described in the literature.[15,16,18,27] A tight Achilles tendon increases pressure on the midfoot, hindfoot, and forefoot. Equinus is caused by glycosylation of the tendon secondary to hyperglycemia. With every procedure, the authors perform either a tendo-achilles lengthening or a gastrocnemius-soleus release; in some instances an Achilles tenotomy is necessary. The purpose is to increase the calcaneal inclination angle and decrease the abnormal pressures that can lead to ulcerations. One must be careful not to overlengthen the tendon, which can lead to a calcaneal gait, increasing the pressures on the heel.

ANKLE ARTHRODESIS

Charcot ankle deformity has an incidence of approximately 10%.[30] The associated instability and progressive deformity result in ulceration in a high number of cases, which can lead to osteomyelitis and amputation (**Fig. 8**). **Fig. 9** shows loss of alignment of the foot and ankle, with protrusion of the lateral or medial malleolus. The authors believe the Charcot ankle deformity is the most challenging to treat both conservatively and surgically, but with advancing technologies in both internal and external fixation, limb salvage is becoming more consistent.[31]

An acute ankle Charcot deformity is less stable and more likely to require surgery. The authors' approach to acute Charcot ankle surgery is similar to the approach they use for the midfoot. In the acute setting the authors are likely to relocate the deformity and apply an external fixator to stabilize the Charcot process. Their standard neutral three-ring fixator is preferred. When evidence of radiographic coalescence is

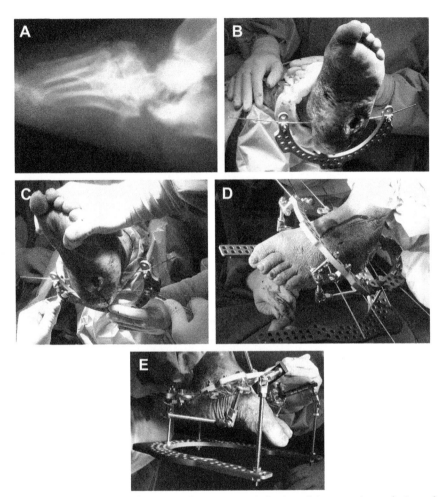

Fig. 7. (*A*) Stage 1 acute Charcot with coexisting infection. (*B*) Bent-wire technique for fusion. (*C*) "Russianing" the wires to provide uniform compression at the arthrodesis site. (*D*) Configuration of a miter frame. (*E*) Completion of miter aspect of frame for tarsal fusion using the bent-wire technique.

present in 2 to 3 months, the external fixator is removed and any corrective osteotomies or ostectomies are performed with the necessary internal fixation. In the presence of a noninfected ulcer, the authors will debride the ulceration and apply the appropriate type of skin graft before applying the external fixator. In the presence of an infected ulceration or osteomyelitis, all necrotic nonviable tissue or bone is resected, antibiotic beads are placed, parental antibiotics are started, and then the external fixator is applied.

For the chronic Charcot stage with deformity, the authors will relocate all necessary joints and apply an external fixator (**Fig. 10**). In approximately 6 weeks the external fixator is removed and internal fixation is applied (**Fig. 11**). If mild deformity is present, then the authors advocate using internal fixation with or without external fixation initially. The Charcot deformity of the ankle usually presents with a significant varus deformity, with significant fragmentation of the medial malleolus and talus.[32] In the

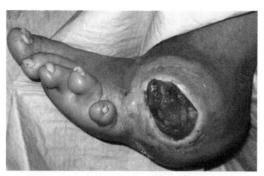

Fig. 8. Severe Charcot ankle deformity with ulceration on the lateral aspect of the ankle.

patient in **Fig. 12**, the authors performed a wedge resection to remove any nonviable and unstable segments of bone. With this technique, they use standard lateral ankle and medial ankle incisions. The lateral incision is used to access the distal portion of the fibula, the subtalar joints, and the calcaneus. The medial incision is used to

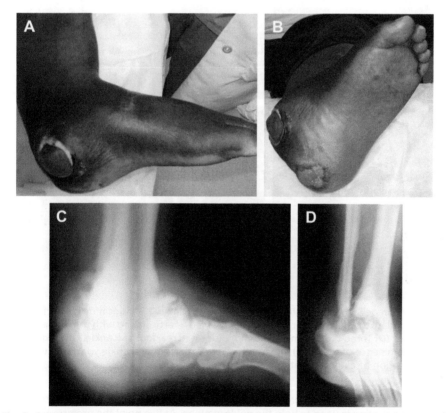

Fig. 9. (*A*) Charcot ankle deformity with ulceration over the medial malleolus. (*B*) Extent of Charcot ankle deformity. (*C*) Lateral radiograph showing destruction of the talus and collapse of the tibia into the calcaneus. (*D*) Anterior-posterior radiograph showing destruction of the ankle joint.

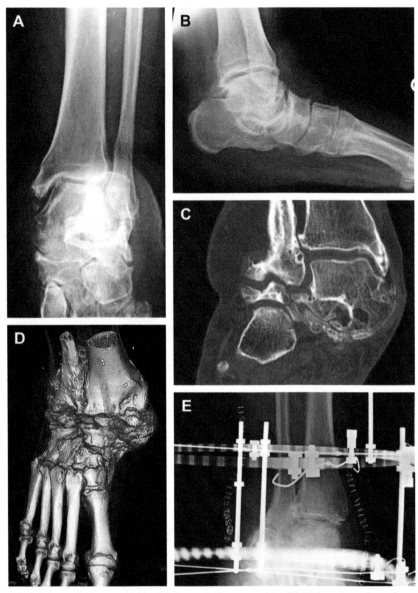

Fig. 10. (*A*) Stage 3 Charcot ankle. (*B*) Stage 3 Charcot ankle. (*C*) Dislocation of rearfoot and ankle secondary to Charcot arthropathy. The calcaneus is articulating with the fibula instead of the talus. (*D*) Three-dimensional CT scan of dislocated rearfoot and ankle, with significant medial prominence of ankle. (*E*) Open reduction of rearfoot and ankle with exostectomies and application of external fixator.

access the medial malleolus and talus. After removal of the wedge, a Steinmann pin or provisional fixation is used to hold the ankle in place. At this point the preferred internal fixation is inserted. The authors prefer to use a compressive intramedullary nail, because they have noticed higher rates of union with this modality. It provides stable compression across the arthrodesis site with adequate rigidity. When an

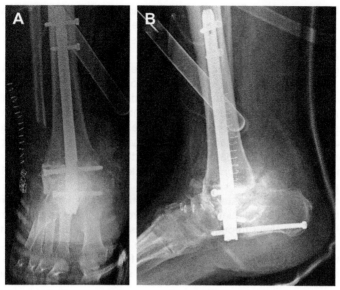

Fig. 11. (*A*) Removal of external fixator and insertion of intramedullary nail with good alignment of rearfoot and ankle. (*B*) Insertion of intramedullary nail for rearfoot and ankle arthrodesis for Charcot stage 3 dislocation.

intramedullary nail cannot be used secondary to plantar ulceration, then locking plates are preferred. The authors do not recommend approaching the Charcot ankle fusion the same way as one would any other ankle fusion. Advanced hardware with compression technology should be used. Simple interfragmentary screws should not be used alone, because the authors' experience has shown that the risk of future failure, recurrence of deformity, or nonunion will increase.

The literature reports mixed results regarding the success of Charcot ankle fusion and satisfaction rates. Eylon and colleagues[33] reviewed 17 patients who underwent an ankle arthrodesis using external fixation alone. All the ankles achieved a solid fusion and the average American Orthopaedic Foot and Ankle Society score was 65 of 86

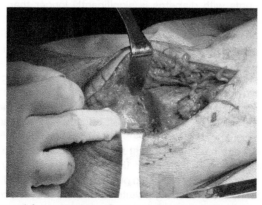

Fig. 12. Wedge removal for correction of varus deformity of the ankle.

possible. The investigators found that the lone Charcot ankle fusion reported the worst possible score. However, they concluded that the Ilizarov technique achieves a high union rate and is especially useful in complex cases, such as revisions and Charcot arthropathy.

Caravaggi and colleagues[34] retrospectively reviewed 14 patients with Charcot late-stage ankle instability who underwent fusion with an intramedullary nail. All ulcerations were healed before surgery. The authors showed a 92.8% salvage rate and 71.4% (10 of 14) solid arthrodesis rate. Moore and colleagues[35] reviewed 19 ankles treated with intramedullary nails for ankle arthrodesis. Most of the patients had Charcot ankle arthropathy with deformity. Five of the seven patients developed a pseudoarthrosis. The investigators concluded that intramedullary nails should be used for salvage, especially in patients with bone loss and osteopenia, such as those with neuroarthropathy.

Pinzur and Kelikian[36] advocated arthrodesis of the subtalar joint using a retrograde intramedullary rodding technique for Charcot arthropathy. They performed retrograde nailing of the subtalar joint through the calcaneus and talus and into the tibia of 21 ankles. Of the 21 ankles, 19 fused at an average of 20 months' follow-up. Recently biomechanical data from one study suggest that fixation with a retrograde, statically locked intramedullary nail may provide the most stable construct for Charcot ankle arthrodesis.[37]

Myerson and colleagues[38] used a blade plate to perform 26 tibiocalcaneal fusions and reported a union rate of 92.3%. This article's authors have used blade plates for ankle fusions in the Charcot population with acceptable results. In the patient in **Fig. 13**, it was used for a revisional ankle fusion after nonunion. Locking plates such as these have great advantages in high-risk patients, and are ideal in osteopenic bone. The authors recommend their use when an intramedullary nail fails or is not suitable option for fixation.

BIOLOGICS

For every high-risk surgical procedure, especially Charcot reconstructive procedures, the authors always use some form of autograft or allograft. The ideal bone substitute to use should possess all three qualities of bone healing: osteogenesis, osteoinductive, and osteoconductive. Some studies have shown a high nonunion rate for Charcot arthrodesis procedures.[39] Loder[40] reported that the overall union rate for fractures was 163% longer in patients with diabetes than in normal controls. The healing time for fractures in patients with diabetes is significantly longer than in those without. Therefore, the authors highly recommend the use of biologics for Charcot reconstructions. Using autograft bone adds to procedure time and possibly increases the chance of a complication. Using a fibular strut when removing the fibula from an ankle arthrodesis procedure is an exception to this. The portion of fibula removed is morselized and used in the arthrodesis procedure. The authors mainly use allograft bone, which contains osteoinductive and osteoconductive properties. Demineralized bone matrix (DBM) is mainly used at Hahnemann University Hospital. DBM is thought to possess more inductive properties than regular allograft because growth factor availability is increased after the demineralization process.[41] Ragni and Lindholm[42] showed that DBM with hydroxyapatite had the quickest fusion rate compared with autograft and DBM or hydroxyapatite. They concluded that these findings may be the result of increased availability of bone morphogenic protein (BMP)–saturated DBM potentiated by the increased connectivity of the graft site. BMPs are proteins found within bone that stimulate mesenchymal cells to differentiate into osteoblasts (osteoinductive

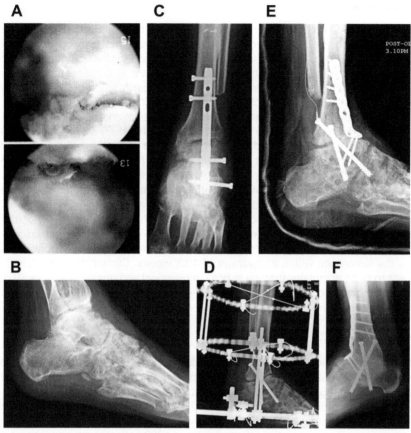

Fig. 13. (A) Arthroscopic view of a Charcot ankle. (B) Stage 3 Charcot of the ankle and rear-foot and midfoot joints. (C) Nonunion of ankle joint status post intramedullary nail. (D) Second attempt of ankle arthrodesis with internal and external fixation. (E) Combination of interfragmentary screws and anterior blade plate for ankle fusion status post external fixator removal. (F) Solid fusion of ankle and subtalar joints with interfragmentary screws and anterior blade plate.

properties).[43] The authors routinely use a high concentration of BMP DBM, called Trel-Xpress 300c (Integra LifeSciences Corporation, Irvine, CA, USA). It contains Accell Bone Matrix (ABM), which is an open-structured dispersed form of DBM, which provides accessibility to bone proteins without the need to be broken down. This dispersed form of DBM increases the surface area, which provides access to natural bone proteins. It also incorporates a poloxamer Reverse Phase Medium, a highly biocompatible carrier. To provide an even better healing environment, the authors mix this DBM with bone marrow aspirate (BMA). BMA is usually harvested from the distal tibia for a midfoot procedure or from the proximal tibia when performing an ankle or more proximal procedure. It is thought that adding BMA to this highly concentrated DBM will provide the osteogenicity property of bone healing. When bigger gaps or voids need to be filled, the authors use fresh frozen allograft, such as femoral head. Femoral head is used most often by the authors when a talectomy is performed and needed for a tibiocalcaneal arthrodesis.

BONE STIMULATION

Bone stimulation devices have been reported as adjunctive therapy in the treatment of Charcot osteoarthropathy. Currently studies are limited but provide encouraging results in patients who are not surgical candidates and those who have undergone reconstructive arthrodesis. One study performed by Hanft and colleagues[44] followed a group of 31 patients with acute stage 1 Charcot osteoarthropathy, all of whom were treated with an offloading protocol of either a total contact cast or a cam walker and limited ambulation. A bone stimulator to be used in conjunction with offloading therapy was also prescribed in 21 of these patients. Results of this study showed a 12.8-week difference in the time for consolidation compared with patients who did not receive bone stimulator therapy. A recent retrospective study preformed in 2005 by Saxena and colleagues[45] followed a population of 26 high-risk patients after arthrodesis procedures with implantation of an electrical bone stimulator device. Inclusion criteria for this patient population included diabetes, body mass index greater then 28, previous history of smoking or alcohol abuse, failed arthrodesis, or a history of immunosuppressive agents, such as steroids. Sixteen of the patients were diagnosed with Charcot osteoarthropathy. Results of this study showed radiographic consolidation across the fusion site within an average of 10.3 weeks. Current literature suggests a benefit to bone stimulator therapy in both the surgical and nonsurgical populations, but larger randomized control studies are needed to further assess the usefulness of bone stimulators in the treatment of patients with Charcot osteoarthropathy.

COMPLICATIONS

Postoperative complications in patients with Charcot osteoarthropathy can be serious and more frequent than in the typical patient population. The most common cause of Charcot osteoarthropathy is uncontrolled diabetes mellitus. Diabetes mellitus is well known to have significantly increased incidence of delayed wound healing and increased infection rates. A retrospective study by Wukich and colleagues[46] published in 2010 compared postoperative infection rates in 1000 patients with and without diabetes mellitus who underwent foot and ankle surgery. Results showed a postoperative infection rate of 13.2% in the diabetic population compared with 2.8% in the nondiabetic population. Further analysis showed that when the neuropathic diabetic population was excluded, no significant difference was seen between the controlled diabetic population and the nondiabetic population. This study indicates a 10-fold increase of infection rates between the nondiabetic population and the neuropathic or uncontrolled diabetic population. This study shows the need for increased attention to compliance and local wound care after surgery in patients with Charcot. Previous authors have suggested an increased incidence of delayed union and nonunion after surgery in patients with Charcot, which may indicate the use of a bone stimulator.[45] Proper attention to and management of these patients is of the upmost importance to maximize potential for a positive outcome.

POSTOPERATIVE CARE

Patients placed in external fixators are kept strictly non–weight-bearing, either with crutches or a wheelchair. The authors are aware that early weight-bearing is an advantage of external fixation, but patients in the urban setting of center city Philadelphia are known for their noncompliance. The authors have rarely seen breakage or loosening of wires or fixators because of this. In the acute phase of Charcot, the authors apply external fixators as a standard. External fixators are removed after bony coalescence is seen on radiographs, which usually occurs 2 to 3 months after the initial surgery. Internal hardware is then inserted and the patient is immobilized in a fiberglass cast for another 8 weeks on average, and is then transitioned into a soft cast with a cam walker for another 4 to 6 weeks. Patients are then casted for custom molded braces, shoes, or orthotics. In the later stages of Charcot deformity, the authors usually use a combination of internal and external fixation. The external fixator is usually removed after 6 weeks. Patients are then placed in a below-knee fiberglass cast for another 8 weeks and then transitioned into a soft cast with a cam walker boot for another 4 to 6 weeks. They are then casted for custom molded braces, shoes, or orthotics. In the senior author's private practice, patients with Charcot who have undergone reconstructive surgery are followed once weekly for the first 3 months, biweekly for the next 2 months, and eventually monthly for follow-up and care. If patients are immobilized for extended periods, than the authors sometimes prescribe alendronate, 35 mg or 70 mg weekly, to prevent disuse osteopenia. When the authors have applied these postoperative principles with meticulous surgical considerations and good surgical technique, they have seen a high rate of union and surgical success and an improvement in patient-reported quality of life.

DISCUSSION

Arthrodesis of the foot and ankle in patients with Charcot can be challenging but also rewarding when the final outcome is successful. The authors strongly believe in using advanced fixation technology to surgically treat the Charcot foot and ankle. In their experience, a combination of internal and external fixation must be used for fusion of the midfoot and ankle in these patients. Advanced biologics and bone stimulators should also be used. Any treatment modalities that will assist in healing are highly recommended. Foot and ankle surgeons should not approach fusions of the Charcot foot the same as they do for primary fusions performed for arthritis. Detailed surgical knowledge and experience are needed for these cases. When following their treatment standards, the authors have noticed an increase in fusion rates and limb salvage.

REFERENCES

1. Anderson LB, DiPreta J. Charcot of the calcaneus. Foot Ankle Clin 2006;11: 825–35.
2. Frykberg R, Belczyk R. Epidemiology of the Charcot foot. Clin Podiatr Med Surg 2008;25:17–28.
3. Jeffcoate W. The causes of the Charcot syndrome. Clin Podiatr Med Surg 2008; 25:29–42.
4. Marks R. Complications of foot and ankle surgery in patients with diabetes. Clin Orthop 2001;391:153–61.
5. Gill G, Hayat H, Maijid S. Diagnostic delays in diabetic Charcot arthropathy. Practical Diabetes International 2004;21(7):261–2.
6. Rogers L, Bevilacqua N. The diagnosis of Charcot foot. Clin Podiatr Med Surg 2008;25:43–51.
7. Eichenholtz SN. Charcot joints. Springfield (IL): Charles C Thomas; 1966. p. 3–10.
8. Yu GV, Hudson JR. Evaluation and treatment of stage 0 Charcot neuroarthropathy of the foot and ankle. J Am Podiatr Med Assoc 2002;92(4):210–20.
9. Sella EJ, Barrette C. Staging of Charcot neuroarthropathy along the medial column of the foot in the diabetic patient. J Foot Ankle Surg 1999;38:34–40.

10. Sanders L, Frykberg R. The Charcot foot. The high risk foot in diabetes mellitus. New York: Churchill Livingstone; 1991.
11. Sella E, Grosser D. Imaging modalities of the diabetic foot. Clin Podiatr Med Surg 2003;20:729–40.
12. Jostel A, Jude E. Medical treatment of Charcot neuroosteoarthropathy. Clin Podiatr Med Surg 2008;25:63–9.
13. Sinacore DR. Acute Charcot arthropathy in patients diabetes mellitus: healing times by foot location. J Diabetes Complications 1998;12(5):287–93.
14. Anderson JJ, Woelffer KE, Holtzman JJ, et al. Bisphosphonates for the treatment of Charcot neuroarthropathy. J Foot Ankle Surg 2004;43(5):285–9.
15. Jolly GP, Zgonis T, Polyzois V. External fixation in the management of Charcot neuroarthropathy. Clin Podiatr Med Surg 2003;20:741–56.
16. Hamilton GA, Ford LA. External fixation of the foot and ankle Elective indications and techniques for external fixation in the midfoot. Clin Podiatr Med Surg 2003; 20:45–63.
17. Simon SJ, Tejwani SG, Wilson DL. Arthrodesis as an early alternative to nonoperative management of Charcot arthropathy of the diabetic foot. J Bone Joint Surg Am 2000;82:939–50.
18. Roukis TS, Zgonis T. The management of acute Charcot fracture-dislocations with the Taylor's spatial external fixation system. Clin Podiatr Med Surg 2006;23:467–83.
19. Papa J, Myerson M, Girard P. Salvage, with arthrodesis in intractable diabetic neuropathic arthropathy of the foot and ankle. J Bone Joint Surg Am 1993;75: 1056–66.
20. Early JS, Hansen ST. Surgical reconstruction of the diabetic foot: a salvage approach for midfoot collapse. Foot Ankle Int 1996;17:325–30.
21. Rooney J, Hutabarat S, Grujic L, et al. Surgical reconstruction of the neuropathic foot. Foot 2002;12:213–23.
22. Assal M, Stern R. Realignment and extended fusion with use of a medial column screw for midfoot deformities secondary to diabetic neuropathy. J Bone Joint Surg Am 2009;91:812–20.
23. Sammarco JV, Sammarco J, Walker EW, et al. Midtarsal arthrodesis in the treatment of Charcot midfoot arthropathy: surgical technique. J Bone Joint Surg Am 2010;92:1–19.
24. Grant WP, Lavin-Garcia S, Sabo R. Beaming the columns for Charcot diabetic foot reconstruction: a retrospective analysis. J Foot Ankle Surg 2011;50:182–9.
25. Sammarco VJ. Superconstructs in the treatment of Charcot foot deformity: plantar plating, locked plating and axial screw fixation. Foot Ankle Clin 2009;14:393–407.
26. Zonno AJ, Myerson MS. Surgical correction of midfoot arthritis with and without deformity. Foot Ankle Clin 2011;16:35–47.
27. Wang JC. Use of external fixation in the reconstruction of the Charcot foot and ankle. Clin Podiatr Med Surg 2003;20:97–117.
28. Pinzur MS. Neutral ring fixation for high-risk nonplantigrade Charcot midfoot deformity. Foot Ankle Int 2007;28(9):961–6.
29. Grant WP, Garcia-Lavin SE, Sabo RT, et al. A retrospective analysis of 50 consecutive Charcot diabetic salvage reconstructions. J Foot Ankle Surg 2009;48(1):30–8.
30. Sticha RS, Franscone ST, Wertheimer SJ. Major arthrodesis in patients with neuropathic arthropathy. J Foot Ankle Surg 1996;35:560–6.
31. Burns PR, Wukich DK. Surgical reconstruction of the Charcot rearfoot and ankle. Clin Podiatr Med Surg 2008;25:95–120.
32. Conway JD. Charcot salvage of the foot and ankle using external fixation. Foot Ankle Clin 2008;13:157–73.

33. Eylon S, Porat S, Bor N, et al. Outcome of Ilizarov ankle arthrodesis. Foot Ankle Int 2007;28(8):873–9.
34. Caravaggi C, Cimmino M, Caruso S, et al. Intramedullary compressive nail fixation for the treatment of severe Charcot deformity of the ankle and rearfoot. J Foot Ankle Surg 2006;45:20–4.
35. Moore TJ, Prince R, Pochatko D, et al. Retrograde intramedullary nailing for ankle arthrodesis. Foot Ankle Int 1995;16(7):433–66.
36. Pinzur M, Kelikian A. Charcot ankle fusion with a retrograde locked intramedullary nail. Foot Ankle Int 1997;18(11):699–703.
37. Mueckley TM, Eichorn S, von Oldenburg G, et al. Biomechanical evaluation of primary stiffness of tibiotalar arthrodesis with an intramedullary compression nail and four other fixation devices. Foot Ankle Int 2006;27:814–20.
38. Myerson M, Alvarez R, Lam P. Tibiocalcaneal arthrodesis for the management of severe ankle and hindfoot deformities. Foot Ankle Int 2000;21(8):643–50.
39. Hockenbury TR, Gruttadauria M, McKinney I. Use of implantable bone growth stimulation in Charcot ankle arthrodesis. Foot Ankle Int 2007;28(9):971–6.
40. Loder RT. The influence of diabetes mellitus on the healing of closed fractures. Clin Orthop 1988;232:210–6.
41. Pacaccio DJ, Stern SF. Demineralized bone matrix: basic science and clinical applications. Clin Podiatr Med Surg 2005;22:599–606.
42. Ragni P, Lindholm TS. Interaction of allogeneic DBM and porous HA bioceramics in lumbar interbody fusion in rabbits. Clin Orthop 1991;272:292–9.
43. Cook EA, Cook JJ. Bone graft substitutes and allografts for reconstruction of the foot and ankle. Clin Podiatr Med Surg 2009;26:589–605.
44. Hanft JR, Goggin JP, Landsman A, et al. The role of combined magnetic field bone growth stimulation as an adjunct in the treatment of neuroarthropathy/Charcot joint: an expanded pilot study. J Foot Ankle Surg 1998;37(6):510–5.
45. Saxena A, DiDomenico LA, Widtfeldt A, et al. Implantable electrical bone stimulator for arthrodesis of the foot and ankle in high-risk patients: a multicenter Study. J Foot Ankle Surg 2005;44(6):450–4.
46. Wukich DK, Lowery NJ, McMillen RL, et al. Postoperative infection rates in foot and ankle surgery: a comparison of patients with and without diabetes mellitus. J Bone Joint Surg Am 2010;92(2):287–95.

Current Concepts and Techniques in Foot and Ankle Surgery

First Metatarsophalangeal Joint Arthrodiastasis and Biologic Resurfacing with External Fixation: A Case Report

Crystal L. Ramanujam, DPM, MSc, Steven Kissel, DPM,
Alex Stewart, DPM, Thomas Zgonis, DPM*

KEYWORDS

• Hallux rigidus • Biologics • Metatarsophalangeal joint
• External fixation • Arthrodiastasis

Symptomatic degenerative arthritis of the first metatarsophalangeal joint (MTPJ), which encompasses a range of presentations from hallux limitus to hallux rigidus, has a variety of causes including previous osteochondral injury, biomechanical alterations, and inflammatory conditions.[1] Early symptoms include pain, swelling, and stiffness in the joint with forced dorsiflexion, such as with walking, running, squatting, toe raises, or simply with passive range of motion. The patient may present with difficulty wearing shoes, especially those that require dorsiflexion of the first MTPJ, such as high heels. Advancing symptoms of hallux rigidus are noted when the patient has almost constant pain at the joint, possibly even at rest. Joint crepitus is also noted with progressing symptoms because of the formation of joint osteophytes or destruction of the articular surfaces. Enlarging osteophytosis can lead to a visible and palpable osseous mass, typically at the dorsal aspect of the joint. Depending on the severity, difficulty walking may lead to transfer metatarsalgia, as well as knee pain, hip pain, or back pain caused by patients altering their gate patterns to attempt to alleviate the strain on the first MTPJ.[2] The early stages of hallux rigidus are usually amenable to conservative treatment, whereas later stages often require surgical

Division of Podiatric Medicine and Surgery, Department of Orthopaedic Surgery, University of Texas Health Science Center at San Antonio, 7703 Floyd Curl Drive–MSC 7776, San Antonio, TX 78229, USA
* Corresponding author.
E-mail address: zgonis@uthscsa.edu

Clin Podiatr Med Surg 29 (2012) 137–141
doi:10.1016/j.cpm.2011.10.003
0891-8422/12/$ – see front matter © 2012 Elsevier Inc. All rights reserved.

intervention. Concomitant hallux abducto valgus deformity can compound the clinical scenario and requires careful consideration in surgical planning. Recent surgical advances have led to numerous joint-sparing options for this painful and debilitating disorder. This article presents a case illustrating an innovative surgical technique for hallux rigidus through aggressive joint debridement combined with first MTPJ biologic resurfacing and arthrodiastasis.

CASE REPORT

A 64-year-old woman presented with a painful left first MTPJ after previously undergoing a distal first metatarsal osteotomy with screw fixation for correction of hallux abducto valgus deformity. The patient was otherwise healthy. Her primary symptoms included pain both with activity and at rest, swelling, and limited range of motion at the first MTPJ. Radiographs of the foot showed significant narrowing of the first MTPJ, recurrent hallux valgus with intact screw fixation, and lateralization of the sesamoids. After a lengthy discussion of continued conservative measures versus surgical correction, the patient elected to proceed to surgery based on her activity level and functional expectations.

Under general anesthesia and pneumatic thigh tourniquet, a linear incision was created at the dorsal aspect of the first MTPJ followed by deep dissection to expose the joint. The first metatarsal head screw was located and removed. The metatarsal head and proximal phalangeal base were debrided of any remaining osteophytes and the articular cartilage at the first metatarsal head was inspected as the joint was distracted. Articular damage at the plantar distal aspect of the first metatarsal head was visualized and a 0.045 Kirschner wire was used for subchondral drilling. Next, a 5 cm by 5 cm collagen-glycosaminoglycan monolayer graft (Integra Lifesciences, Plainsboro, NJ, USA) was then carefully placed directly over the first metatarsal head extending proximally to the metatarsal neck. Any excess graft was resected appropriately and 5 mL of fibrin sealant was applied to secure the graft in place. The surgical site was then closed in layered fashion. The tourniquet was deflated and a new sterile field was set up about the foot for placement of the uniplane monolateral external fixation device (Stryker Hoffmann External Fixation System, Mahwah, NJ, USA). Under fluoroscopic guidance, three 3-mm half pins were inserted from medial to lateral direction: the first pin at the midpoint of the medial cuneiform, the second pin at the first metatarsal base 1 cm distal to the articular surface, and the third pin at the base of the proximal phalanx of the hallux. The monolateral external fixator was assembled with appropriate clamps followed by a long carbon fiber rod. Manual distraction and positioning of the first metatarsal was achieved while the external fixation device was secured by appropriate tightening. Intraoperative C-arm fluoroscopy was used to confirm maintained distraction at the first MTPJ. Once the construct was noted to be stable, dry sterile dressings followed by a well-padded posterior splint was applied to the lower extremity. The patient maintained partial weight bearing status to the left foot for 6 weeks, with biweekly clinic visits for serial radiographs and evaluation of incisions/pin sites. The external fixator was removed at approximately 6 weeks and the patient progressed to full weight bearing status with passive and active range of motion exercises to the first MTPJ. At 9 months' follow-up, the patient was pain free and able to maintain her active lifestyle (**Fig. 1**).

DISCUSSION

Many factors such as joint space, intra-articular cartilage damage, periarticular osteophytosis, sesamoid function, and complete ankylosis of the joint should be assessed

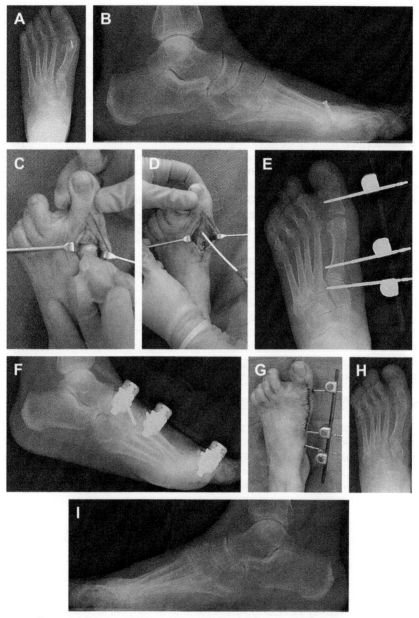

Fig. 1. Radiographic anteroposterior (*A*) and lateral (*B*) views of the left foot showing the recurrent hallux abducto valgus deformity and associated first MTPJ disorder with narrowing and arthritic changes. Intraoperative views of the collagen-glycosaminoglycan monolayer at the first MTPJ (*C*) secured by the application of a fibrin sealant (*D*) after extensive joint debridement and removal of the internal screw fixation. Postoperative radiographic (*E, F*) and clinical views (*G*) showing the application of the uniplane monolateral external fixation system for the first MTPJ arthrodiastasis procedure. Postoperative radiographic views (*H, I*) at approximately 9 months' follow-up.

when planning any joint salvage procedure for treatment of hallux rigidus. When performing first MTPJ reconstruction, the first step is surgical removal of any associated joint osteophytes and the releasing of any restrictive adhesions about the joint. One of the simplest, effective, and most traditional method of cartilage repair is subchondral drilling with microfracture of the subchondral bone.[3] This technique involves multiple perforations in the subchondral bone to stimulate and maintain the body's natural healing processes in an attempt to promote fibrocartilage formation at the defect. Although hyaline cartilage formation is optimal for replacement of the degenerative areas, fibrocartilage repair can also offer relief of arthritic symptoms.[4]

Further surgical techniques have been described with the insertion of an interposing membrane to resurface and replace the arthritic joint's cartilage. Some of the earliest described procedures used materials such as chromicized porcine bladder, cellophane, and nylon.[2] Autogenous interposing membranes such as the fascia lata, dermal graft, and full-thickness skin graft have also been described in detail.[2] The use of a collagen-glycosaminoglycan monolayer as the joint interposing membrane eliminates donor site morbidity and reduces the risk of host immune response to the inserted graft.[2,4,5] Furthermore, arthrodiastasis is a helpful adjunctive procedure that facilitates intermittent increases in joint pressures and offloads the joint surfaces.[6] In the absence of mechanical stress, these changes in joint pressure are hypothesized to cause a corresponding increase in proteoglycan synthesis that promotes hyaline cartilage repair. Arthrodiastasis has been reported to be useful in delaying the need for arthrodesis in cases of moderate to severe degenerative arthritis.[7–9]

The combination of surgical procedures performed in this case provided deformity correction and resolution of symptoms while avoiding the need for immediate joint-destructive procedures. These surgical techniques allow preservation of anatomy so that future surgical procedures may be considered, if warranted.

SUMMARY

Numerous surgical options exist for the treatment of hallux rigidus, depending on the stage and severity at clinical presentation. This article presents an alternative approach for salvaging the first MTPJ by combining a first MTPJ arthrodiastasis and biologic resurfacing. Careful patient selection and knowledge of external fixation are necessary for a successful patient outcome.

REFERENCES

1. Schnirring-Judge M, Hehemann D. The cheilectomy and its modifications. Clin Podiatr Med Surg 2011;28:305–27.
2. Brigido S, Troiano M, Schoenhaus H. Biologic resurfacing of the ankle and first metatarsophalangeal joint: case studies with a 2-year follow-up. Clin Podiatr Med Surg 2009;26:633–45.
3. Steadman J, Rodkey W, Rodrigo J. Microfracture: surgical technique and rehabilitation to treat chondral defects. Clin Orthop Relat Res 2001;391:362–9.
4. Rubin L, Schweitzer S. The use of acellular biologic tissue patches in foot and ankle surgery. Clin Podiatr Med Surg 2005;22:533–52.
5. Berlet G, Hyer C, Lee TH, et al. Interpositional arthroplasty of the first MTP joint using a regenerative tissue matrix for the treatment of advanced hallux rigidus. Foot Ankle Int 2008;29:10–21.
6. Zgonis T, Stapleton JJ, Roukis TS. Use of circular external fixation for combined subtalar joint arthrodesis and ankle distraction. Clin Podiatr Med Surg 2008;25: 745–53.

7. Aldegheri R, Trivella G, Saleh M. Articulated distraction of the hip. Conservative surgery for arthritis in young patients. Clin Orthop Relat Res 1994;301:94–101.
8. van Roermund PM, Marijnissen AC, Lafeber FP. Joint distraction as an alternative for the treatment of osteoarthritis. Foot Ankle Clin 2002;7:515–27.
9. Ramanujam CL, Sagray B, Zgonis T. Subtalar joint arthrodesis, ankle arthrodiastasis, and talar dome resurfacing with the use of a collagen-glycosaminoglycan monolayer. Clin Podiatr Med Surg 2010;27:327–33.

Surgical Soft Tissue Closure of Severe Diabetic Foot Infections: A Combination of Biologics, Negative Pressure Wound Therapy, and Skin Grafting

Crystal L. Ramanujam, DPM, MSc, Thomas Zgonis, DPM*

KEYWORDS

- Diabetic foot • Wounds • Neuropathy • Biologics
- Negative pressure wound therapy • Amputation

Foot infections and associated wounds are the leading cause of hospitalization of diabetics.[1] Expedited closure of diabetic foot wounds can reduce the risk for major limb amputation and decrease costs associated with prolonged wound care.[2] Well-established surgical techniques such as primary closure, flaps, and skin grafting are not always suitable for early closure of extensive diabetic foot and ankle wounds. Recent advances in wound care modalities, including tissue-engineered products such as bilayer matrix scaffolds, can accelerate healing in these patients.[3] The Integra Bilayer Matrix Wound Dressing (Integra Life Sciences, Plainsboro, NJ, USA) is a collagen-based synthetic graft that facilitates cellular invasion and capillary growth into the wound, and its outer layer is made from silicone. The adjunctive use of negative pressure wound therapy (NPWT) can augment the healing process and prepare for definitive closure through skin grafting. This article presents a stepwise approach detailing the combination of these surgical techniques for the closure of complicated diabetic foot wounds.

Division of Podiatric Medicine and Surgery, Department of Orthopaedic Surgery, University of Texas Health Science Center at San Antonio, 7703 Floyd Curl Drive-MSC 7776, San Antonio, TX 78229, USA
* Corresponding author.
E-mail address: zgonis@uthscsa.edu

Clin Podiatr Med Surg 29 (2012) 143–146
doi:10.1016/j.cpm.2011.10.004
0891-8422/12/$ – see front matter © 2012 Elsevier Inc. All rights reserved.

CASE REPORT

A 53-year-old diabetic man presented to the emergency room for treatment of left foot pain, redness, and swelling. A rock had fallen on it 3 days before. He initially self-treated the injury by soaking the foot in hot salt water, but noticed worsening redness of the entire foot and ankle. He denied constitutional symptoms on presentation. His past medical history was positive for uncontrolled diabetes mellitus and hypertension and he was noncompliant with outpatient medications.

General physical examination revealed a well-nourished, Spanish-speaking man in no acute distress. Vital signs showed an increased blood pressure but absence of fever or tachycardia. Foot and ankle examination showed palpable pedal pulses with pitting edema and cellulitis extending from the level of the toes to the ankle. Full-thickness ulceration was located at the medial aspect of the fourth digit with probing to deep soft tissues, serosanguinous drainage, and severe sloughing of necrotic skin on the entire toe. Small superficial ulcerations were found at the medial aspect of the fifth digit and lateral third digit. The patient also had leukocytosis and severe hyperglycemia. Radiographs of the foot and ankle revealed subcutaneous emphysema at the fourth digit. Based on the clinical and radiographic findings, the patient was admitted for urgent surgical intervention. He was medically optimized and cleared by the medicine team, and consented for left foot debridement to the level of an open partial fourth ray amputation. The initial surgical procedure consisted of aggressive debridement, cultures of bone and soft tissue, and open partial fourth ray amputation. He was maintained on intravenous broad-spectrum antibiotics with revisional surgery 4 days later for soft tissue debridement and NPWT device placement because of the depth of the remaining surgical wound defect. The patient was discharged to home on culture-specific oral antibiotics following normalization of laboratory values and no further evidence of clinical infection.

Five weeks later, after undergoing local wound care 3 times weekly for NPWT dressing changes, the wound depth had significantly decreased without recurrence of infection. Because of the large length and width of the surgical wound, the patient was brought back to the operating room for surgical application of Integra Bilayer Matrix Wound Dressing to promote further epithelialization. Surgical wound bed preparation to stimulate healthy bleeding tissue was performed via hydrosurgical debridement. The Integra Bilayer Matrix Wound Dressing was moistened in sterile saline and meshed in a 1:1 fashion to allow wound drainage and prevent fluid accumulation beneath the graft. The graft was then secured to the wound with staples, with the silicone layer facing away from the wound bed and with the graft well adhered to the wound surface with minimal tension. NPWT (VAC, Kinetic Concepts Inc., San Antonio, TX, USA) was also applied over the biologic wound bilayer to enhance incorporation during the early healing phase. Subsequent intraoperative wound cultures at this time were negative and the patient had removal of the NPWT device in the outpatient setting within the following 8 days. The patient was then transitioned to a non–weight-bearing lower extremity posterior splint for an additional 3 weeks and subsequent staple removal.

Eight weeks later, and after local wound care with moist to dry dressings, the patient returned to the operating room for definitive wound closure through split thickness skin grafting (STSG). The recipient wound bed was first prepared through hydrosurgical debridement. The donor site at the lower lateral aspect of the ipsilateral leg was used for the skin harvesting. An electric dermatome was used to carefully harvest the appropriately sized skin graft, which was meshed in a 1:1.5 ratio. The harvested STSG was anchored to the recipient bed by staples followed by application of a bolster dressing and a well-padded lower extremity posterior splint. After 3 weeks of non–weight bearing to the operative foot, the dressing and staples were removed revealing great healing signs at both the recipient and donor sites. The patient was then transitioned to full weight-bearing status in a postoperative shoe and eventually progressed into extra depth shoes. At the patient's latest clinical visit at 18 weeks, he had no recurrence of wound or infection and no difficulty with ambulation (**Fig. 1**).

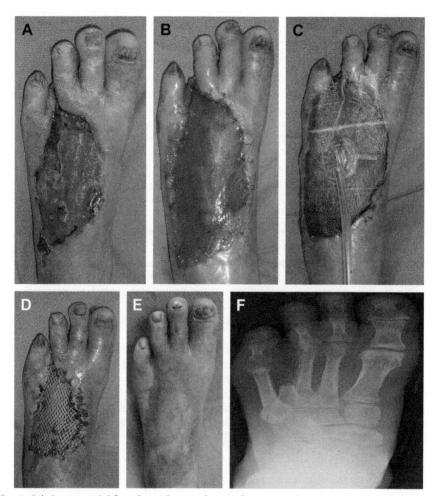

Fig. 1. (*A*) Open partial fourth ray (toe and part of metatarsal) amputation showing extensive soft tissue defect from a severe diabetic foot infection. Patient underwent hydrosurgical debridement with application of an Integra Bilayer Matrix Wound Dressing (Integra Life Sciences, Plainsboro, NJ, USA) (*B*) that was secured by a NPWT device (VAC, Kinetic Concepts Inc., San Antonio, TX, USA) (*C*). The NPWT was removed at 8 days and the patient followed a regimen of local wound care, appropriate off-loading and oral antibiosis for approximately 11 weeks. The patient then returned to the operating room for a definitive wound closure with an autogenous split thickness skin graft (*D*). Postoperative clinical (*E*) and radiographic (*F*) outcomes with complete wound closure at approximately 18 weeks' follow-up.

DISCUSSION

Local wound care and off-loading continue to provide the standard of care for diabetic wounds without infection. Prolonging definitive closure of the diabetic wound has the potential to lead to recurring infection and risks further amputation.[4] The option of advanced biologic wound materials is advantageous because of the ease of the technique and the ability to use local anesthesia with a shorter duration of surgery.[5] In addition, the use of NPWT has long been established as a reliable and cost-effective modality for wound closure.[6] This method consistently provides a moist healing environment while removing unwanted exudates from the wound bed, and can effectively promote adherence of grafts to the recipient wound base. In addition, STSG provides closure of wounds in a simple manner associated with shorter healing times and lower cost compared with other wound healing modalities.[7]

SUMMARY

For complicated diabetic foot wounds resulting after initial debridement of severe infections, rapid definitive closure can often elude even the most experienced surgeon. Along with a multidisciplinary approach to controlling infection and optimizing overall medical status, the authors encourage the creative use of techniques readily available on the reconstructive armamentarium. Aggressive surgical debridement and consecutive application of NPWT, biologics, and STSG can provide long-term functional wound closure in the diabetic patient.

REFERENCES

1. Reiber GE, Lipsky BA, Gibbons GW. The burden of diabetic foot ulcers. Am J Surg 1998;176(Suppl 2A):5–10.
2. Ramsey SD, Newton K, Blough D, et al. Incidence, outcomes, and cost of foot ulcers in patients with diabetes. Diabetes Care 1999;22(3):382–7.
3. Collier M. The use of advanced biological and tissue-engineered wound products. Nurs Stand 2006;21(7):68–76.
4. Capobianco CM, Stapleton JJ, Zgonis T. Soft tissue reconstruction pyramid in the diabetic foot. Foot Ankle Spec 2010;3:241–8.
5. Ramanujam CL, Capobianco CM, Zgonis T. Using a bilayer matrix wound dressing for closure of complicated diabetic foot wounds. J Wound Care 2010;19:56–60.
6. Clemens MW, Broyles JM, Le PN, et al. Innovation and management of diabetic foot wounds. Surg Technol Int 2010;20:61–71.
7. Roukis TS. Skin grafting techniques for open diabetic foot wounds. In: Zgonis T, editor. Surgical reconstruction of the diabetic foot and ankle. Philadelphia: Lippincott Williams & Wilkins; 2009. p. 129–39.

Index

Note: Page numbers of article titles are in **boldface** type.

Clin Podiatr Med Surg 29 (2012) 147–154
doi:10.1016/S0891-8422(11)00124-8
0891-8422/12/$ – see front matter © 2012 Elsevier Inc. All rights reserved.

podiatric.theclinics.com

Printed and bound by CPI Group (UK) Ltd, Croydon, CR0 4YY

03/10/2024

01040444-0007

Moving?

Make sure your subscription moves with you!

To notify us of your new address, find your **Clinics Account Number** (located on your mailing label above your name), and contact customer service at:

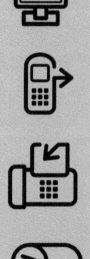

Email: **journalscustomerservice-usa@elsevier.com**

800-654-2452 (subscribers in the U.S. & Canada)
314-447-8871 (subscribers outside of the U.S. & Canada)

Fax number: **314-447-8029**

Elsevier Health Sciences Division
Subscription Customer Service
3251 Riverport Lane
Maryland Heights, MO 63043

*To ensure uninterrupted delivery of your subscription, please notify us at least 4 weeks in advance of move.

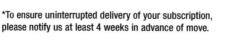